JN234683

日本医学英語教育学会・編

講義録
医学英語 Ⅰ

語彙の充実と読解力の向上

編集　清水雅子（川崎医療福祉大学教授）

Textbook of
English for
Medical Purposes
Volume I
Building Vocabulary and Reading Comprehension

MEDICAL VIEW

Textbook of English for Medical Purposes, Volume 1
Building Vocabulary and Reading Comprehension
(ISBN 978-4-7583-0407-8 C3347)

Edited by Masako Shimizu for the Japan Society for Medical English Education

2005. 1.20 1st ed.

©MEDICAL VIEW, 2005
Printed and Bound in Japan

Medical View Co., Ltd.
2-30 Ichigaya-hommuracho, Shinjuku-ku, Tokyo 162-0845, Japan
E-mail ed@medicalview.co.jp

刊行に寄せて

　本書は，医師・医療関係者に求められる英語力を総合的・体系的に習得するための全3巻の教科書として，日本医学英語教育学会により企画・編集されました。

　かねてから医師には英語力も必要だと言われていたものの，医師・医学生への英語教育は「医学」と「英語教育」という2つの異なる専門分野での知識が要求され，体系的に教育できるカリキュラムや教材もないまま，現場で担当する先生たちは独自の工夫をこらしつつ大変な努力をなさっていました。日本医学英語教育学会が1998年に設立された際には，その大きな目的の一つとして，この2つの分野の専門家たちが協力することによって，日本における医学英語教育の指針となるべき教科書を制作することがありました。爾来6年，その努力が実を結んだ成果が本書です。

　本書を企画段階において，医師に求められる英語力の到達目標として下記の3点が挙げられました。

1. 英語で患者さんの診療を行える。
2. 英語で医療・医学に関する発表・討論を行える。
3. 英語で論文や書類を作成できる。

　最終的にこれらの目標に到達するためのステップとして，本書の各章は構成されています。全3巻は英語力の段階に応じて分けられており，初級向けの第1巻では語彙の充実や読解力の養成を，第2巻では医学の専門的内容にさらに踏み込んで症例報告や論文を題材として採り上げ，第3巻では実践の準備段階として，患者さんとの会話や口頭発表，論文執筆について学びます。

　言うまでもなく，外国語の習得に王道はありません。学生の間だけで上記の到達目標に到達するのは難しいかもしれませんが，卒業して医師となってからも，生涯続く英語学習の友として本書を活用していただければ，これに勝る喜びはありません。

　現在のわが国は，残念ながら諸外国からの評価としては「医学・医療知識の輸入国」としての地位に甘んじています。しかし前途有望な医師・医学生の皆さんが本書を学習の友として英語力の研鑽に励まれれば，その汚名を返上できる日も遠くはないと確信しています。

2004年12月

日本医学英語教育学会理事長
東京慈恵会医科大学脳神経外科教授

大井 静雄

序文

　20年以上前のことです。私は「医学英語教育の現状を語ろう」というバロン先生(現・日本医学英語教育学会副理事長)の呼びかけに関心をもち，直接お電話をしましたが，あいにく先生はお留守でした。先生にお会いしたのは，その10年余後，多くの医学教育者と英語教育者が集まった日本医学英語教育研究会でした。研究会はさほど年月を要することなく学会へと成長しました。それは，医学生の英語力養成に悪戦苦闘する医学と英語の両教育分野の教師達が，植村研一先生(初代理事長)の「国際的に通用する英語運用能力をもつ医師養成」への情熱に共鳴したためと思われます。

　この度の3巻から成る『講義録　医学英語』の刊行が，立場の異なる学会員たちの活動が結実したものであることは，現理事長の大井静雄先生が「刊行に寄せて」に記しているとおりです。本書，第1巻は「基本語彙と読解力の育成」を目ざし，学習者が医学英語には初級者であることを考慮して，以下のように構成しました。

Chapter 1	日本の医療制度の特徴（英文と語彙）
Chapters 2～5	基礎的な語彙（語彙の構成要素と体系別身体語彙）
Chapters 6～8	ニュース番組から（糖尿病，自閉症，SARS，心疾患）
Chapters 9～12	医療の現場で使う英語表現
	（会話形式による医学・医療表現の習得）

　各章には，学習内容の理解を深めるために詳細な説明を加え，学習を確実にするために練習問題を付しています。

　医学英語運用能力の基礎である専門語彙は，一種の記号とみなして丸暗記していく学習方法もあります。けれどもそれは膨大な医学語彙数を記憶するには，効果的な方法とは言えません。ここでは徐々に，けれども確実に語彙学習の"こつ"を習得します。

　英文読解力の養成は，医療に身近な内容の英文や実際に診療に用いる会話体を，聞く・書く・発声することと併せて学習できるように構成しました。

　言語習得には短期的な集中学習と，気の遠くなるような長期学習とを必要とします。また，実際にその言語を使えるようになるには，日本語運用能力や人としての総合力をも必要とします。典型的な英語表現を覚えても，内容がなければ空疎な自己表現に留まってしまうでしょう。本書が，伝えるべきメッセージを持つ医師を目指す第一歩となることを祈っております。

　最後に，本書の発刊にあたって編集・校正にご尽力をいただきました，日本医学英語教育学会事務局担当の江口潤司様に，心よりお礼申しあげます。

2004年12月

『講義録　医学英語I』編集委員
日本医学英語教育学会理事
川崎医療福祉大学英語教授

清水 雅子

Contents

刊行に寄せて … iii
序文 …………… iv
編集委員会 …… x

Part 1　Medical System in Japan

Chapter 1　Characteristics of the Medical System in Japan　　2

The System by which Doctors are Qualified and Permitted to Open Offices Freely ———————————————————— 2
The Free Choice System for Patients ———————————— 3
Medical Care Insurance System for Everyone ——————— 4

Part 2　Medical Terminology

Chapter 2　Medical Terminology (1)　　10

法則を見つけよう ———————————————————— 12
■ 意味を共有する接尾辞を見つけよう … 12
■ 'o' に注目 … 13

Chapter 3　Medical Terminology (2)　　16

基本的な接尾辞を覚えよう ———————————————— 16
■ –algia … 16
■ –itis … 17
■ –osis … 18
■ –oma … 19

連結形を変化させよう —————————————————— 20
■ gastr–（胃）＋他の要素 … 20
■ cardi–（心臓）＋他の要素 … 21
■ 複雑な構造の語の要素 … 22

Chapter 4　Medical Terminology (3)　　26

連結母音と構成要素の組合せ：4つの鉄則 ————————— 26
鉄則❶と❷の組合せ ——————————————————— 27
鉄則❸ ————————————————————————— 29
鉄則❹ ————————————————————————— 30

例外 ─────────────────────────────── 31
- ■ 語根が2つ以上ある例 … 31
- ■ 接頭辞の最後の母音を取らない例 … 32
- ■ 特定の個人の名前からつくられた用語 … 32

Chapter 5　Body Parts　　　　　　　　　　　　　　　　34

External Body Parts　身体の外面 ─────────── 34
- ■ head　頭 … 34
- ■ face　顔 … 34
- ■ neck　頸，首 … 34
- ■ trunk　体幹 … 35
- ■ extremities　四肢 … 35

Musculoskeletal System　筋骨格系 ──────────── 37
- ■ bone　骨 … 37
- ■ muscle　筋肉 … 38

Blood & Immune System　血液・免疫系 ─────────── 40
- ■ heart　心臓 … 40
- ■ blood vessels　血管 … 40
- ■ blood　血液 … 40
- ■ lymph　リンパ … 41

Respiratory System　呼吸器系 ────────────── 42

Digestive System　消化器系 ───────────────── 44
- ■ oral cavity　口腔 … 44
- ■ stomach　胃 … 44
- ■ small intestine　小腸 … 45
- ■ large intestine　大腸 … 45

Urinary System　泌尿器系 ──────────────── 47

Endocrine System　内分泌系 ──────────────── 48

Reproductive System (Genital System)　生殖器系 ──────── 49
- ■ male genital organs　男性生殖器 … 49
- ■ female genital organs　女性生殖器 … 49

Nervous System　神経系 ──────────────── 51
- ■ brain　脳 … 51
- ■ central nervous system　中枢神経系 … 52

Sensory Organs　感覚器官 — 54
- visual organ　視覚器官 … 54
- auditory organ　聴覚器官 … 55

Skin　皮膚 — 56

Miscellaneous　その他 — 57

Part 3　Listening to Medical News

Chapter 6　Listening to Medical News (1)　60
Silent Killer — 60
Autism: Early Signs — 64

Chapter 7　Listening to Medical News (2)　68
Coping with SARS in the U.S. — 68
Caring for the First SARS Patient in the U.S. — 72

Chapter 8　Listening to Medical News (3)　76
Heart Test — 76
Growing Arteries — 79

Part 4　Learning Medical Expressions

Chapter 9　Expressions to Describe Signs and Symptoms　84
At an outpatient clinic: A case of digestive problems — 84
After the physical examination — 86
Word Check — 88
- 症状 … 88
- 基本的な医学用語 … 88
- 動詞表現 … 90
- その他 … 90

Word Study ──────────────────────────── **90**
- symptoms と signs の相違は？ … 90
- 「症状」に関する表現 … 91
- 「症状」を表す用語 … 92
- 会話表現 … 93
- 冠詞の用法 … 95
- bring on ...（症状の増悪因子について確認する表現）… 97

Chapter 10　Expressions to Describe Vital Signs　　102

In the ER: Mr. Smith was brought to the ER by ambulance.
　He is suffering from an ongoing chest pain. ──── **102**
After further physical examinations ─────────── **104**
Word Check ──────────────────────────── **106**
- vital signs に関する用語 … 106
- 基本的な医学用語 … 107
- 動詞表現 … 107
- 検査用語 … 107
- その他 … 109

Word Study ──────────────────────────── **109**
- 「胸痛」について … 109
- 「罹っている」の表現 … 109
- 患者さんを落ち着かせる表現 … 110
- 症状がいつから生じたのかを尋ねる表現 … 111
- vital signs をチェックするときの表現 … 111
- 血圧値を英語で読む場合 … 111
- 脈拍数を英語で読む場合 … 112
- 「正常範囲内」という表現 … 112
- 会話で用いられる英単語と医療用語との違い … 112

Chapter 11　Expressions to Describe Pain　　116

A suspected case of angina pectoris ─────────── **116**
After the physical examination ──────────────── **118**

Word Check — 120
- 痛みに関する表現 … 120
- 基本的な医学用語・検査用語 … 120
- 動詞表現 … 120
- 会話表現 … 121
- その他 … 122

Word Study — 122
- 「痛み」の有無を尋ねる表現 … 122
- 「痛み」の存在を訴える … 124

Chapter 12　Expressions to Use in the Examination — 130
Case 1. A patient with bronchitis — 130
Case 2. A patient with a sprained ankle — 132
Word Check — 134
Word Study — 134
- 検査の表現 … 134

Index — 140

COLUMN
- 医学英語にはなぜギリシャ語源とラテン語源が多いのか？
　①ギリシャ語からラテン語へ …… 15
- 日本の医学用語のルーツ …… 23
- 医学英語はどう発音するか？ …… 32
- 杉田玄白と前野良沢 …… 53
- 医学英語にはなぜギリシャ語源とラテン語源が多いのか？
　②ラテン語を仲介したフランス語 …… 67
- 初診の患者さんに相対するときの心得（1）…… 85
- 初診の患者さんに相対するときの心得（2）…… 97
- Vital Signs …… 103
- 癌はなぜカニなのか？ …… 115
- 「痛み」の表現 …… 117
- さまざまな意味をもつ "colic" …… 125

日本医学英語教育学会
医学英語教科書編集委員会

■編集委員会

小林充尚（委員長）	防衛医科大学校名誉教授
大木俊夫	浜松医科大学名誉教授
大武　博	京都府立医科大学第一外国語教室教授
大野典也	東京慈恵会医科大学名誉教授
Nell L. Kennedy	酪農学園大学獣医学部バイオメディカルイングリッシュ研究室教授
清水雅子	川崎医療福祉大学英語教授
羽白　清	元・京都大学
J. Patrick Barron	東京医科大学国際医学情報センター教授
菱田治子	浜松医科大学英語助教授

■第1巻担当編集委員

清水雅子	川崎医療福祉大学英語教授

■第1巻執筆者

安藤千春	獨協医科大学医学部英語助教授（Chapters 2～4）
玉巻欣子	神戸大学医学部非常勤講師（Chapter 5）
森　茂	大分大学医学部英語助教授（Chapters 6～8）
横田眞二	相模台病院腎センター部長（Chapters 9～12）

Part 1
Medical System in Japan

Part 1: Medical System in Japan

Chapter 1: Characteristics of the Medical System in Japan

POINT ☞
1. 日本の医療制度の特徴を学ぼう。
2. 専門科目・専門医の名称を学ぼう。

Reading

The medical system in Japan has three main characteristics. First, doctors and dentists who receive their national license can open their own offices if they so desire. Second, patients can choose the medical care facilities from which they wish to receive treatment. Third, all residents are, in principle, required to take part in some form of medical care insurance.

facility: 施設，設備
treatment: 治療，処置
medical care insurance:
　医療保険，健康保険

The System by which Doctors are Qualified and Permitted to Open Offices Freely

Licensing is available nationwide for doctors and dentists. They can work anyplace they desire if they have satisfactory contract conditions, and they can open their own clinic or hospital if they have the capital required. (It is necessary for them to report their intentions to open an office and in certain cases to receive permission from the local administration.) In areas where the number of beds per hospital is over the standard set by Medical Law, however, increasing the number of beds has not been officially permitted since the end of the 1980's.

Medical Law: 医事法

To become a doctor in Japan, a person must complete six years in a medical department of a university and must then pass the national examination given by the Japanese government (the Ministry of Health, Labour and Welfare). On passing the examination, the person is licensed as a doctor, but many doctors go on for two years or more of training. After that, the doctor either works in a hospital or opens his/her own office. Once licensed, the doctor is allowed to treat any illness, but most doctors will specialize in a specific area of treatment. Some doctors will change their area of specialization after undergoing further training and carrying out research.

In Japan, there is no system by which the government authorizes specialist licenses for doctors. However, there is a system by which each of the academic circles in medicine (such as internal medicine, surgery, neurosurgery, pediatrics, etc.) give specialist certifications. The standard of qualification varies from circle to circle, however, and doctors are not supposed to advertise that they are qualified as specialists. This principle also goes for dentists. Nearly all nurses and other medical related personnel take part in a public licensing system.

The Free Choice System for Patients

Under the second characteristic, patients living anywhere in Japan can receive treatment at any clinic or hospital. Most hospitals have an outpatient department, so persons seeking treatment can go directly to the hospital without having to go to a clinic or private doctor

national examination: 国家試験

the Ministry of Health, Labour and Welfare: 厚生労働省

specialize in ...: …を専攻する

internal medicine: 内科学

surgery: 外科学

neurosurgery: 脳神経外科学

pediatrics: 小児科学

outpatient department: 外来部門

first. However, it is common for patients with only mild complaints to be disallowed to choose a specific doctor to provide treatment at large hospitals. Proper treatment can depend on the type of illness, the person's everyday living conditions, and the physical condition of the person at the time of treatment; therefore, it is recommended that you find a doctor or dentist that you can trust, who lives nearby and who you can consult with confidence. When necessary a doctor or dentist will refer a patient to the proper hospital or to another clinic for treatment.

complaint: 不平，病訴
（< complain:〔病苦を〕訴える）

Medical Care Insurance System for Everyone

In Japan, since 1961, citizens have, in principle, been obliged to take part in one of the public medical care insurance systems. At present, this includes all residents, except international patients who are staying in Japan only for a short period.

The exception to this is those persons who are given the opportunity to apply for public assistance (seikatsuhogo) because of their limited income. Necessary medical treatment is guaranteed them under the public assistance system. This system is also applicable to the international community.

Since almost 100% of the residents in Japan take part in some form of public medical care insurance, almost 100% of the medical care facilities use the public medical care insurance to cover the cost of treatment.

As you can probably guess, medical care facilities which do not participate in the public medical care insurance system are unusual, amounting to a limited number of special clinics. Under this system, one can go to any medical organization and expect to receive the same treatment for the same cost as anywhere else. However, hospitals and clinics are ranked a little differently under the public medical care insurance system. There are also various fees such as the first examination fee, or re-examination fee, so even if one receives the same treatment, depending on the time required and the place, there might be a difference in the fee.

examination: 検査，診察

Reprinted with permission from the Webpage "Medical Care and Public Health in Kitakyushu" (http://www.city.kitakyushu.jp/~k1003030/medical/medical1e.html).

Comprehension Check

・日本の医療制度における3つの特徴は何ですか。日本語で答えなさい。

_____

_____

_____

Further Study

1. 諸外国における医療制度を調べて，日本の制度と比較してみましょう。

_____

_____

_____

2. 専門科目と専門医の名称を覚えましょう。

doctor; physician [fɪzíʃən] ; practitioner [præktíʃ(ə)nɚ]	医師
attending physician	主治医，担当医
general practitioner (GP); family doctor; primary physician	一般開業医，家庭医
intern [íntɚːn, ɪntéːn]	インターン，医学研修生
resident [rézədnt]	レジデント，研修医
specialist	専門医
anesthesiology [æ̀nəsθìːziálədʒi]	麻酔科〔学〕
anesthesiologist; anésthetist	麻酔医
cardiology [kɑ̀ːdiálədʒi]	心臓〔病〕学
cardiologist; heart doctor	心臓〔病〕学者，心臓専門医
dentistry [déntɪstri]	歯科〔学〕
dentist	歯科医
dermatology [dɚ̀ːmətálədʒi]	皮膚科〔学〕
dermatologist; skin specialist	皮膚科医
endocrinology [èndəkrɪnálədʒi]	内分泌〔学〕
endocrinologist	内分泌学者
gastroenterology [gæ̀strouentərálədʒi]	胃腸病科〔学〕
gastroenterologist	胃腸病学者
geriatrics [dʒèriǽtrɪks]; gerontology [dʒèrəntálədʒi]	老年医学，老人医学，老年病学
geriatrician; gerontologist	老年医学者
gynecology [gàɪnəkálədʒi, dʒìnə-]	婦人科〔学〕
gynecologist	婦人科医
hematology [hìːmətálədʒi]	血液〔病〕学
hematologist	血液〔病〕学者
internal medicine	内科〔学〕
internist [íntɚːnɪst]; physician	内科医

neurology [n(j)urálədʒi]	神経内科〔学〕；神経〔科〕学
neurologist; brain specialist	神経内科医；神経〔科〕学者
neurosurgery [n(j)ùrousə́:rdʒəri]	脳神経外科〔学〕
neurosurgeon	脳神経外科医
obstetrics [əbstétrɪks, ɔ-]	産科〔学〕
obstetrician [àbstetríʃən, ɔ-]	産科医
oncology	腫瘍学
oncologist	腫瘍学者
ophthalmology [àfθælmálədʒi]	眼科〔学〕
ophthalmologist; eye doctor	眼科医
orthopedics [ɔ̀:rθəpí:dɪks]	整形外科〔学〕
orthopedist	整形外科医
oto〔rhino〕laryngology [òutou〔ràinou〕lærɪŋgálədʒi]	耳鼻咽喉科〔学〕
oto〔rhino〕laryngologist; ENT doctor	耳鼻咽喉科医
（ENT は ear, nose and throat の頭文字）	
pediatrics [pì:diǽtrɪks]	小児科〔学〕
pediatrícian; children's doctor	小児科医
plastic surgery	形成外科〔学〕
plastic surgeon	形成外科医
psychiatry [sikáɪətri, sɑi-]	精神科〔学〕
psychiatrist	精神科医
radiology [rèɪdiálədʒɪ]	放射線科〔学〕
radiologist	放射線科医
surgery	外科〔学〕
surgeon [sə́:rdʒən]	外科医
urology [juərálədʒi]	泌尿器科〔学〕
urologist	泌尿器科医

Part 2
Medical Terminology

Part 2: Medical Terminology

Chapter 2 Medical Terminology (1)

> **POINT** ☞ 医学用語の成り立ちの法則を学ぼう。

Lecture

　医学用語（英語）はいくつくらいあるのでしょうか。言葉は刻々と創られては消えていくものですから，厳密な数は不明です。いちおう辞書に掲載されている用語を「定着しているもの」と考えて判断するしかありません。

　現在日本で出版されている代表的な医学辞典をみると，A社の医学辞典には10万語，B社には23万語，C社には15万語が収録されています。それにしても膨大な数です。もちろん，皆さんが将来これをすべて使用するわけではなく，自分の専門領域で用いる用語はそのなかの一部に限られるでしょうが，そうはいってもかなりの数に及ぶでしょう。

　また，初めて医学英語に接する人は，英語のような英語でないような単語にとまどうことが多いでしょう。それも当然です。なぜなら，医学用語には英語そのもののほかに，フランス語を経由してギリシャ語やラテン語が英語に同化されたものが，きわめて多いからです。しかしこのことによって，むしろ医学英語の習得が簡単になるということをこれから説明します。

　以下に医学用語をいくつかあげてみました。なかには皆さんがこれまでに見聞きしたことのある単語もあると思います。知っている単語には印を付けてみましょう。

- ☐ adenoid
- ☐ allergy
- ☐ anesthetic
- ☐ anemia
- ☐ antitoxin
- ☐ appendicitis
- ☐ arteriosclerosis
- ☐ aspirin
- ☐ bacteriology
- ☐ bronchitis
- ☐ bronchoscope
- ☐ carbohydrate
- ☐ cholesterol
- ☐ clinic
- ☐ diphtheria
- ☐ endocrine gland
- ☐ enzyme
- ☐ homeopathic
- ☐ hormone
- ☐ immunology
- ☐ insulin
- ☐ iodine
- ☐ metabolism
- ☐ morphine
- ☐ orthodontia
- ☐ osteoporosis
- ☐ penicillin
- ☐ protein
- ☐ stethoscope
- ☐ streptomycin
- ☐ vaccinate

日本語では順に，

- ☐ アデノイド
- ☐ アレルギー
- ☐ 麻酔
- ☐ 貧血
- ☐ 抗毒素
- ☐ 虫垂炎
- ☐ 動脈硬化
- ☐ アスピリン
- ☐ 細菌学
- ☐ 気管支炎
- ☐ 気管支鏡
- ☐ 炭水化物
- ☐ コレステロール
- ☐ クリニック
- ☐ ジフテリア
- ☐ 内分泌腺
- ☐ 酵素
- ☐ 同種療法の
- ☐ ホルモン
- ☐ 免疫学
- ☐ インスリン
- ☐ ヨウ素
- ☐ 代謝
- ☐ モルヒネ
- ☐ 歯科矯正学
- ☐ 骨粗鬆症
- ☐ ペニシリン
- ☐ 蛋白
- ☐ 聴診器
- ☐ ストレプトマイシン
- ☐ 予防接種（ワクチン接種）する

「習うより慣れろ」とも言います。けれども膨大な数の単語を一つ一つ丸暗記していくのは，時間と労力の無駄にすぎません。効率よく習得するには，用語を構成する基本法則を知っておくと便利です。まずはコツを会得しましょう。

法則を見つけよう

■意味を共有する接尾辞を見つけよう

手始めに，前項で列挙した用語から，同じ語尾をもつものを選んでみましょう．

1) anestheti<u>c</u>　　　【*adj.*】麻酔の；【*n.*】麻酔薬
   clini<u>c</u>　　　　　クリニック，臨床講義
   homeopathi<u>c</u>　　同種療法の
2) anem<u>ia</u>　　　　　貧血
   diphther<u>ia</u>　　　ジフテリア
   orthodont<u>ia</u>　　歯科矯正〔学〕
3) antitox<u>in</u>　　　抗毒素
   aspir<u>in</u>　　　　アスピリン
   insul<u>in</u>　　　　インスリン
   prote<u>in</u>　　　　蛋白
   penicill<u>in</u>　　　ペニシリン
   streptomyc<u>in</u>　　ストレプトマイシン
4) appendic<u>itis</u>　　虫垂炎
   bronch<u>itis</u>　　　気管支炎
5) bacterio<u>logy</u>　　細菌学
   immuno<u>logy</u>　　　免疫学
6) broncho<u>scope</u>　　気管支鏡
   stetho<u>scope</u>　　　聴診器
7) carbohydr<u>ate</u>　　炭水化物
   vaccin<u>ate</u>　　　　予防接種する

日本語訳を参考にすると，多くの語が接尾辞(–ic，–ia，–in，–itis，–logy，–scope，–ate)によって同じような意味をもつグループに分類されていることがわかるでしょう．逆に，例えば bronchitis と bronchoscope を比べてみれば，接尾辞 –itis と –scope によって語根(bronch–)の意味が変化することが理解できるでしょう．そこで導き出される法則は，

> 法則1：接尾辞はその前の部分に個別の意味を与える。

■ 'o' に注目

　分類した語を別の視点から見ると，あることに気づくでしょう。前項の5) と6) では，接尾辞の直前に 'o' があります。この 'o' がある語とない語を要素に分けて比べてみましょう。

　bronchitis　→　bronch/itis（気管支/炎症）
　bronchoscope　→　bronch/o/scope（気管支/o/鏡）

'o' には意味がないことがわかります。けれども，前項で列挙した単語から 'o' があるものを選んでみると，結構多いのです。

　adenoid, arteriosclerosis, bacteriology, bronchoscope, carbohydrate, endocrine, homeopathic, immunology, metabolism, orthodontia, osteoporosis, stethoscope, streptomycin

　これらを 'o' に着目して見ると，adenoid と osteoporosis 以外は 'o' の前後が子音であること，そして 'o' は意味ある部分である語根の間に位置していることがわかるでしょう。そこで，

> 法則2　'o' は意味ある語根をつなぐ働きをする。
> 法則3　'o' は子音と子音をつなぐ働きをする。

　ただし，adenoid は aden/oid（腺/のような）という単独の意味をもつ -oid の一部です。このように母音がすでに含まれている場合は，adenooid とは重ねません。また，osteoporosis は oste/o/porosos と，oste に母音が含まれていてもなぜか 'o' を挿入します。これは子音と子音の間に 'o' を入れるこ

とと同様に，osteporosis よりも 'o' を入れて oste**o**porosis とするほうが発音するときに都合がよいためだと考えられます。この 'o' を文法用語で「連結母音」とよびます。母音は 'o' に限る必要はないはずですが，'o' を用いることが圧倒的に多いのです。連結母音については Chapter 4 で改めて説明を加えます。

以上の法則 1～3 と，前に説明した接頭辞（anemia の an- 等）を併せてまとめると，医学用語（英語）はほぼ次のように構成されています。

> 医学用語＝接頭辞＋語根（＋連結母音 'o'）＋接尾辞

それでは，これらの構成要素を定義しておきましょう。

- **語根**（**word root**）：用語の核となる要素。他の構成要素が付加され，より複雑な語をつくる。医学用語の場合は，身体の部位を意味するものが多い。
- **接頭辞**（**prefix**）：語根を修飾する要素。名称が表すように，語根の前に付く。通常，位置や数を意味する。
- **接尾辞**（**suffix**）：語根を修飾する要素。名称が表すように，語根の最後に付く。通常，状態を意味する。
- **連結母音**（**combining vowel**）：これ自体に意味はないが，接尾辞を語根に接続したり，語根と語根をつなぐときに使用する。連結母音の大部分はアルファベットの 'o' である。（語根＋連結母音の形を連結形［combining form］と呼ぶ。）

このように，医学用語はステレオタイプな接頭辞，接尾辞と多彩な連結形によって構成されるのですから，これらの基礎的な知識をもつことが，皆さんの頭脳に医学辞書をつくっていく早道となるでしょう。

COLUMN

医学英語にはなぜギリシャ語源とラテン語源が多いのか？ ①ギリシャ語からラテン語へ

　皆さんが医学英語の勉強で最も頭を痛めるのは，これまで学んだ英語とスペリングの形や長さがかなり違っている点でしょう。この医学英語特有の性質を理解するためには，英語の歴史を知る必要がありそうです。

　ヒポクラテスは，医師を目指す人の倫理綱領である Hippocratic Oath（ヒポクラテスの誓い）で必ず出会う，医師の模範となった人です。しかし，ギリシャ時代には，彼ばかりでなく，哲学者ソクラテス，その弟子プラトン，数学のアルキメデス等々，私たちに馴染み深い偉大な学者・知識人が，西洋文明の礎であるギリシャ文明を形成しました（1000 B.C.頃）。その当時の共通ギリシャ語が，アレキサンダー大王の征服によって地中海東部の共通言語となり，同時にギリシャ文明も各地に伝えられたのでした。その後，ヨーロッパは強大なローマ帝国（27 B.C.～395）の支配に置かれ，その政治的影響力とともにローマ人の言語であったラテン語が各地に普及することになりました。

　しかし，それはギリシャ文明最盛期からあまり時を隔てていなかったために，ラテン語の中にギリシャ語の影響を大きく受けたことばが残ったのです。

　こうして混じり合ったギリシャ語とラテン語が，北方ヨーロッパの低地ゲルマン語を祖先とする英語にどうやって入っていったかは，次のコラムで紹介しましょう。

（→67頁のCOLUMNへ続く）

Part 2: Medical Terminology

Chapter 3 Medical Terminology (2)

POINT ☞ 前章での学習をもとに，実際に医学用語を分析してみよう。

Lesson

基本的な接尾辞を覚えよう

以下は，語根がほとんど身体の部位を意味し，接尾辞がその状態を意味する最も単純な構成要素からなる用語です。

■ **–algia** [-ǽldʒə]

1. **gastralgia (gastr / algia)**

語根：	gastr	胃
接尾辞：	algia	～痛
意味：	胃の痛みなので「胃痛」	

2. **neuralgia (neur / algia)**

語根：	neur	神経〔組織〕，神経系
接尾辞：	algia	～痛
意味：	神経の痛みなので「神経痛」	

3. **nephralgia (nephr / algia)**

語根：	nephr	腎〔臓〕
接尾辞：	algia	～痛
意味：	腎臓の痛みなので「腎臓痛」	

4. **arthralgia (arthr / algia)**

　　語根：　　　arthr　　　　関節
　　接尾辞：　　algia　　　　〜痛
　　意味：　　　関節の痛みなので「関節痛」

5. **dermatalgia (dermat / algia)**

　　語根：　　　dermat　　　皮膚の
　　接尾辞：　　algia　　　　〜痛
　　意味：　　　皮膚の痛みなので「皮膚痛」

■ **–itis** [-áɪtɪs]

1. **gastritis (gastr / itis)**

　　語根：　　　gastr　　　　胃
　　接尾辞：　　itis　　　　　炎症
　　意味：　　　胃の炎症なので「胃炎」

2. **neuritis (neur / itis)**

　　語根：　　　neur　　　　神経〔組織〕，神経系
　　接尾辞：　　itis　　　　　炎症
　　意味：　　　神経の炎症なので「神経炎」

3. **nephritis (nephr / itis)**

　　語根：　　　nephr　　　腎〔臓〕
　　接尾辞：　　itis　　　　　炎症
　　意味：　　　腎臓の炎症なので「腎炎」

4. **arthritis (arthr / itis)**

　　語根：　　　arthr　　　　関節
　　接尾辞：　　itis　　　　　炎症
　　意味：　　　関節の炎症なので「関節炎」

5. **dermatitis (dermat / itis)**

　　語根： 　　dermat 　　　皮膚の
　　接尾辞： 　itis 　　　　　炎症
　　意味： 　　皮膚の炎症なので「皮膚炎」

■ **–osis** [-óusɪs]

1. **neurosis (neur / osis)**

　　語根： 　　neur 　　　　神経〔組織〕，神経系
　　接尾辞： 　osis 　　　　〔病的〕状態
　　意味： 　　神経症，ノイローゼ

2. **sclerosis (scler / osis)**

　　語根： 　　scler 　　　　堅い
　　接尾辞： 　osis 　　　　〔病的〕状態
　　意味： 　　硬化症

3. **psychosis (psych / osis)**

　　語根： 　　psych 　　　　心
　　接尾辞： 　osis 　　　　〔病的〕状態
　　意味： 　　精神病

4. **asbestosis (asbest / osis)**

　　語根： 　　asbest 　　　　石綿
　　接尾辞： 　osis 　　　　〔病的〕状態
　　意味： 　　石綿症

5. **stenosis (sten / osis)**

　　語根： 　　steb 　　　　狭い
　　接尾辞： 　osis 　　　　〔病的〕状態
　　意味： 　　狭窄〔症〕

–asis, –esis, –iasis も –osis と同じ意味です（例：emesis 嘔吐）。これらは①非炎症性の疾患，②異常な症状，③物質によって発症する疾患，に用いられます。

■ **–oma** [-óumə]

1. **carcinoma (carcin / oma)**
   語根： carcin 癌
   接尾辞： oma 腫，瘤
   意味： 癌，癌腫

2. **sarcoma (sarc / oma)**
   語根： sarc 肉
   接尾辞： oma 腫，瘤
   意味： 肉腫

3. **myoma (my / oma)**
   語根： my 筋肉
   接尾辞： oma 腫，瘤
   意味： 筋腫

4. **hematoma (hemat / oma)**
   語根： hemat 血液
   接尾辞： oma 腫，瘤
   意味： 血腫

5. **hepatoma (hepat / oma)**
   語根： hepat 肝臓
   接尾辞： oma 腫，瘤
   意味： 肝癌，ヘパトーム

その他，疾患や症状を表す接尾辞には，–ia（anemia：貧血），–pathy（neuropathy：神経障害），–agra（podagra：足部痛風）などがあります。

連結形を変化させよう

■ gastr-(胃)＋他の要素

1. **gastric (gastr / ic)**

語根：	gastr	胃
接尾辞：	ic	〜の，〜のような，〜の性質の，〜からなる
意味：	胃の，胃部の，胃のような形の	

2. **gastroenterology (gastr / o / enter / o / logy)**

語根：	gastr	胃
連結母音：	o	
語根：	enter	腸
連結母音：	o	
接尾辞：	logy	ことば，話，論，学問
意味：	胃腸病学	

3. **hypogastric (hypo / gastr / ic)**

接頭辞：	hypo	下に，以下，少しく
語根：	gastr	胃
接尾辞：	ic	〜の，〜のような，〜の性質の，〜からなる
意味：	下腹部の	

4. **gastroduodenitis (gastr / o / duoden / itis)**

語根：	gastr	胃
連結母音：	o	
語根：	duoden	十二指腸
接尾辞：	itis	炎症
意味：	胃十二指腸炎	

■ cardi-(心臓)＋他の要素

1. cardiogram (cardi / o / gram)
語根：　　　cardi　　　心臓
連結母音：o
接尾辞：　　gram　　　記録，図，文書
意味：　　　心拍〔動〕曲線

2. electrocardiogram (electr / o / cardi / o / gram)
語根：　　　electr　　　電気，電解，電子
連結母音：o
語根：　　　cardi　　　心臓
連結母音：o
接尾辞：　　gram　　　記録，図，文書
意味：　　　心電図

3. cardiomyopathy (cardi / o / my / o / pathy)
語根：　　　cardi　　　心臓
連結母音：o
語根：　　　my　　　　筋肉
連結母音：o
接尾辞：　　pathy　　　苦痛，感情，感応，〜症，〜療法
意味：　　　心筋症

4. epicardium (epi / cardi / um)
語根：　　　epi　　　　上の
語根：　　　cardi　　　心臓
接尾辞：　　um　　　　状態を表す
意味：　　　心外膜

■ 複雑な構造の語の要素

次に，単純な構成要素からなる用語に限定せずに，いくつか分析してみましょう。

1. encephalomyelocele

    (en / cephal / o / myel / o / cele)

    接頭辞： en　　　中，内
    語根： cephal　　頭
    連結母音： o
    語根： myel　　髄，脊髄，骨髄
    連結母音： o
    接尾辞： cele　　～の腫瘍，～のヘルニア
    意味： 脳脊髄瘤

2. encephalomeningopathy

    (en / cephal / o / mening / o / pathy)

    接頭辞： en　　　中，内
    語根： cepahl　　頭
    連結母音： o
    語根： mening　　脳膜，髄膜
    連結母音： o
    接尾辞： pathy　　苦痛，～症，～病
    意味： 脳髄膜障害

3. thrombophlebitis (thromb / o / phleb / itis)

    語根： thromb　　血栓
    連結母音： o
    語根： phleb　　静脈
    接尾辞： itis　　炎症
    意味： 血栓静脈炎

4. **polyradiculoneuropathy**

   (poly / radicul / o / neur / o / pathy)

接頭辞：	poly	多くの，複
語根：	radicul	神経根
連結母音：	o	
語根：	neur	神経〔組織〕，神経系
連結母音：	o	
接尾辞：	pathy	苦痛，〜症
意味：		多発〔神経〕根神経障害

以上のように医学用語を分析してみると，要は「組合せ」であることが漠然と理解できるようになったと思います。医学用語は以下の構成要素の組み合わせによってつくられています。

医学用語の 5 つの組合せ

① 語根＋接尾辞
② 語根＋連結母音＋接尾辞
③ 語根＋連結母音＋語根＋接尾辞
④ 語根＋連結母音＋語根＋連結母音＋接尾辞
⑤ 接頭辞＋上記の組合せ

COLUMN

日本の医学用語のルーツ

英語と日本語を比較してみると，同じ用語であっても日本語訳では時に慣用によって短縮されてしまったり，あるいはヒネリが効いているものもあります。（「肝臓炎」ではなく「肝炎」，あるいは「電心図」ではなく「心電図」等）

日本初の医学的解剖は，1754 年に京都の刑場で実施されました。漢方医であった山脇東洋はこれを基に，中国の五臓六腑説を否定する『蔵志』を著しました。その後，蘭方医であった杉田玄白は，1771 年に江戸で刑死者の解剖に立ち会い，その際に西洋の解剖図が正確なことにとても驚き，中川淳庵，前野良沢とともに翻訳したのが，『解体新書』です。このときに，現在でも，そして今後もおそらく未来永劫に使用されるであろう「神経」や「軟骨」という言葉がつくられました。

Practice

　では，これまでに得た知識を頼りに，用語を分析し意味を類推する練習をしてみましょう。

【練習】以下の用語を構成要素に分け，それぞれの要素の意味から類推して訳してみましょう。（正解は次頁）

1. **arteriosclerosis**
   _____
   _____

2. **neuropathy**
   _____
   _____

3. **psychoneurosis**
   _____
   _____

4. **macrocephalia**
   _____
   _____

【正解】

1. **arteri/o/scler/osis**

    語根： arteri　　　動脈
    連結母音：o
    語根： scler　　　堅い
    接尾辞： osis　　　病的状態
    意味： 動脈硬化〔症〕（パターンの③）

2. **neur/o/pathy**

    語根： neur　　　神経組織，神経系
    連結母音：o
    接尾辞： pathy　　　苦痛，感情，感応，〜症，〜療法
    意味： 神経障害，神経病質，ニューロパシー（パターンの②）

3. **psych/o/neur/osis**

    語根： psych　　　霊魂，精神，心理
    連結母音：o
    語根： neur　　　神経組織，神経系
    接尾辞： osis　　　病的状態
    意味： 精神神経症（パターンの③）

    - 接尾辞 –osis の意味は「病的状態」ですが，慣用的に「〜症」と訳すことが圧倒的に多いです。

4. **macr/o/cephal/ia**

    語根： macr　　　異常に大きい，長い
    連結母音：o
    語根： cephal　　　頭
    接尾辞： ia　　　病気の状態
    意味： 大頭蓋症（パターンの③）

    - この用語の接尾辞– ia も上と同様に「〜症」と訳します。

「もう医学英語なんて怖くない」の心境になればしめたものです。

Part 2: Medical Terminology

Chapter 4　Medical Terminology (3)

> **POINT** ☞　連結母音の組合せの基本原則を学ぼう。

Lecture

連結母音と構成要素の組合せ：4つの鉄則

　前章まで，医学用語の構成要素の意味を考えながら，用語を斜線で分け，意味を理解する練習をしました．その途中で，連結形（語根＋連結母音）が最も重要な要素であることを説明しました．ここでは，連結母音を使用するときと使用しないときの基本原則を紹介します．

4つの鉄則─連結母音と構成要素の組合せ

❶ 連結母音は，語根と語根を結ぶときと接尾辞を語根に結ぶときだけに使用します．接頭辞を語根に結びつけるときには決して使用しません．

❷ 接尾辞を語根に結びつけるときは，接尾辞の先頭が子音の場合のときだけに使用します．接尾辞の先頭が母音の場合は，連結母音は使用しません．

❸ 語根と語根を結びつけるときは，常に連結母音を使用します．

❹ 接頭辞を語根に結びつけるときには，連結母音は決して使用しません．ただし，接頭辞の最後が母音で終わり，結びつける先の語根の先頭が母音で始まる場合は，接頭辞の最後の母音を削り落として語根に結びつけます．

鉄則❶と❷の組合せ

1. oophor / itis

語根： oophor 卵巣

接尾辞： itis 炎症

意味： 卵巣炎

- この用語では，接尾辞を語根に結ぶために，連結母音が使われていません。接尾辞が母音で始まるからです。

2. oophor / o / plasty

語根： oophor 卵巣

連結母音： o

接尾辞： plasty 形成外科

意味： 卵巣形成〔術〕

- この用語では，接尾辞と語根を結ぶために連結母音が使われています。接尾辞が子音で始まるからです。

3. angi / oid

語根： angi 血管，リンパ管

接尾辞： oid 〜のような〔もの〕，〜状の〔もの〕

意味： 血管様の

- 接尾辞が母音で始まるので，連結母音は不要です。ここで重要なことがあります。皆さんの中には，語根の最後が母音なので，接尾辞の先頭と含めて，母音が2つ並んでもよいのかと疑問を持たれる方がいるかもしれません。しかし，その心配は不要です。接尾辞を語根に結びつける際には，接尾辞の先頭が母音なのか，子音なのかに着目するだけでよいのです。

4. angi / o / tomy

語根： angi 血管，リンパ管

連結母音： o

接尾辞： tomy 切除，切開〔術〕

意味： 血管切開〔術〕

5. **enter / al**

   語根：　　　enter　　　　腸

   接尾辞：　　al　　　　　～の〔ような〕，～に適した

   意味：　　　腸内の，経腸的な

6. **enter / o / spasm**

   語根：　　　enter　　　　腸

   連結母音：　o

   接尾辞：　　spasm　　　痙攣，発作

   意味：　　　腸痙攣

7. **prostat / ism**

   語根：　　　prostat　　　前立腺

   接尾辞：　　ism　　　　状態，作用，特性，病的状態

   意味：　　　前立腺症

8. **prostat / o / rrhea**

   語根：　　　prostat　　　前立腺

   連結母音：　o

   接尾辞：　　rrhea　　　排出，放出，流出

   意味：　　　前立腺漏

9. **aort / ectasia**

   語根：　　　aort　　　　大動脈

   接尾辞：　　ectasia　　　膨張，拡張

   意味：　　　大動脈拡張〔症〕

10. **aort / o / pexy**

    語根：　　　aort　　　　大動脈

    連結母音：　o

    接尾辞：　　pexy　　　固定

    意味：　　　大動脈胸骨固定術

鉄則❸

1. **oophor / o / cyst / osis**

    語根： oophor 卵巣

    連結母音：o

    語根： cyst 胆嚢，膀胱，嚢胞，包嚢

    接尾辞： osis 〔病的〕状態

    意味： 卵巣嚢腫形成

    ● 語根と語根を結ぶ際には，迷わず連結母音を使ってください。

2. **omphal / o / phleb / itis**

    語根： omphal 臍，臍の緒

    連結母音：o

    語根： phleb 静脈

    接尾辞： itis 炎症

    意味： 臍静脈炎

3. **pancreat / o / duoden / o / stomy**

    語根： pancreat 膵〔臓〕の

    連結母音：o

    語根： duoden 十二指腸

    連結母音：o

    接尾辞： stomy 開口術

    意味： 膵十二指腸吻合〔術〕

4. **ureter / o / lith / o / tomy**

    語根： ureter 尿管

    連結母音：o

    語根： lith 石

    連結母音：o

    接尾辞： tomy 切除，切開〔術〕

    意味： 尿管切石術

5. lept / o / mening / itis

　語根：　　lept　　　　　細かい，薄い
　連結母音：o
　語根：　　mening　　　脳膜，髄膜
　接尾辞：　itis　　　　　炎症
　意味：　　軟膜炎

鉄則❹

1. end / ophthalm / itis

　接頭辞：　end〔o〕　　　内〔部〕の
　語根：　　ophthalm　　　眼
　接尾辞：　itis　　　　　炎症
　意味：　　眼内炎

　● 接頭辞につながる語根が母音で始まっているので，接頭辞の最後の母音を削り落とします。

2. dys / men / o / rrhea

　接頭辞：　dys　　　　　変質，異常，困難
　語根：　　men　　　　　月経〔期間〕
　連結母音：o
　接尾辞：　rrhea　　　　排出，放出，流出
　意味：　　月経困難症

3. hyper / cholesterol / emia

　接頭辞：　hyper　　　　向こうの，超越，超過，過度に
　語根：　　cholesterol　コレステロール，コレステリン
　接尾辞：　emia　　　　 血症
　意味：　　高コレステロール血〔症〕

4. anti / gen / ic

　接頭辞：　anti　　　　　反対の
　語根：　　gen　　　　　 生じる，もたらす

接尾辞： ic 　　　〜の
意味： 抗原性の

5. **hyp / arteri / al**
接頭辞： hyp〔o〕 　下に，以下，少し
語根： arteri 　　動脈
接尾辞： al 　　　〜の〔ような〕
意味： 動脈下の
- 語根が母音で始まるので接頭辞の最後の母音が削られています。

例外

■語根が2つ以上ある例

1. **en / cephal / o / myel / o / neur / o / pathy**
脳脊髄神経障害

2. **en / cephal / o / myel / o / radicul / o / pathy**
脳脊髄神経根障害

3. **ot / o / rhin / o / laryng / o / logy**
耳鼻咽喉科学

4. **psych / o / neur / o / immun / o / logy**
精神神経免疫学

5. **splen / o / myel / o / malac / ia**
脾骨髄軟化〔症〕

なお encephal は，接頭辞＋語根としましたが，1つの語根として考える場合もあります。また，語根の中には接尾辞として使用できるものもありますし，逆に接尾辞が語根として使用される場合もあります。鉄則の例外としては，以下のよ

うなものもあります。

■接頭辞の最後の母音を取らない例
1. **hemi / arthr / o / plasty**
    半関節形成〔術〕

■特定の個人の名前からつくられた用語
1. **pasteurization**
    低温殺菌
    - フランスの細菌学者 Louis Pasteur [1822 〜 95] から。

2. **roentgenograph**
    X 線（レントゲン）撮影
    - ドイツの物理学者 Wilhelm K. Roentgen [1845 〜 1923] から。

COLUMN

医学英語はどう発音するか？

　そろそろ医学英語に慣れてきた皆さんが困っていることがあるとすれば，それは発音ではないでしょうか？一見英語らしくない単語がたくさんありますが，それでも英語の一つなのですから，特殊な発音方法はありません。ところが，一般的な辞書に掲載されている用語は少なく，また医学辞典に掲載されている発音記号はというと，これまで馴染んだ万国発音記号と違っています。日本の医学辞典の多くが，米国で出版された辞書で使われている発音記号を踏襲しているからです。

　そこで，知恵を授けましょう。日本語っぽい発音でも，第 1 アクセントさえ間違えなければ，ネイティブスピーカーに伝わります。では第 1 アクセントの場所は？というと，ほとんどは接尾辞の先頭，あるいは接尾辞直前の連結母音にあるのです。接尾辞の先頭が母音ならそこが，接尾辞の先頭が子音ならその直前の連結母音が第 1 アクセントというわけです。（もちろん例外はありますが…）

Part 2: Medical Terminology

Chapter 5 Body Parts

POINT ☞ 身体の部位名を習得しよう。

Lesson

External Body Parts　身体の外面

■ **head**　　　　　　　　頭

■ **face**　　　　　　　　顔

　forehead　　　　　　　額，前額部

　temple　　　　　　　　こめかみ，側頭部

　ear　　　　　　　　　　耳

　glabella　　　　　　　　眉間

　eyebrow　　　　　　　　眉

　eyelid　　　　　　　　　瞼（まぶた），眼瞼（がんけん）

　eyelash　　　　　　　　まつ毛，睫毛（しょうもう）

　eye　　　　　　　　　　目

　cheek　　　　　　　　　頬（ほお）

　jaw　　　　　　　　　　顎（あご）

　chin　　　　　　　　　　顎先，おとがい

■ **neck**　　　　　　　　頸，首

　nape　　　　　　　　　項（うなじ）

　Adam's apple　　　　　喉仏，喉頭隆起
　(= laryngeal prominence)

Further Study
形容詞形も覚えよう！

facial: 顔の

temporal: 側頭の

cervical: 頸部の

Chapter 5 Body Parts

■ **trunk** 体幹

  chest (= thorax) 胸〔部〕，胸郭
    shoulder 肩
    breast 胸（胸郭の前表面），乳房
    nipple 乳頭
  abdomen ([俗] belly; tummy) 腹部
    navel (= umbilicus) 臍（へそ）
  side (= flank) わき腹
  lower back 腰
    hip 腰（腰の突出部）
  buttocks 臀部
  genital area 陰部
  groin (= inguinal area) 鼠径部（そけいぶ）

■ **extremities** 四肢

  armpit (= axilla) 脇の下；腋窩（えきか）
  upper arm (= brachium) 上腕，二の腕
  forearm (= antebrachium) 前腕
  elbow 肘（ひじ）
  hand 手
  palm 手掌，てのひら
  finger 指
    thumb (= pollex; first finger) 親指
    index finger (= forefinger; second finger) 人さし指
    middle (third) finger 中指
    ring (fourth) finger 薬指
    little (fifth) finger 小指
  wrist 手首
  leg 下肢（かし）

> **Further Study**
> 形容詞形も覚えよう！

abdominal: 腹部の

umbilical: 臍の

thigh (= femur)	大腿(だいたい)
knee	膝(ひざ)
shin	脛(すね)
calf	ふくらはぎ
ankle	足首
instep	足の甲
heel	踵(かかと)
foot (*pl.* feet)	足
sole	足底
the arch of the foot	土踏まず
toe	足指，趾
cf. first toe; big toe	母趾

Exercise

● 文章の中で身体の部位名を覚えよう。

太字の日本語に相当する英語を記入し，英文を完成しなさい。

1) Fever, generalized headache, vomiting, and _____ _____ are common to many types of meningitis.

   熱，頭全体の頭痛，嘔吐，そして<u>首の**硬直**</u>は多くの型の髄膜炎に共通した症状である。

2) In the case of angina pectoris, chest pain may radiate to the shoulder, neck, or _____ .

   狭心症の場合，肩や首または<u>**腹部**</u>に胸痛が広がっていくことがある。

3) _____ _____ is the most common malignancy among women.

   <u>**乳がん**</u>は女性の間で最も頻度の高い悪性のがんである。

4) The _____ and hands form a complex unit of small, highly active joints used almost continuously during waking hours.

手首と手は，覚醒している間絶え間なく使われる小さくて大変活発に動く関節が複雑に集まってできている。

5) Despite thick padding along the toes, _____ , and heel and stabilizing ligaments at the ankles, the ankle and foot are frequent sites of sprain and bony injury.

足指，足裏，そしてかかとに分厚いクッションがあり，足首にはそれを支える靭帯があるにもかかわらず，足首と足は捻挫や骨の怪我がよく起こる場所である。

6) Angiography in the arterial system from the abdomen to the _____ showed no abnormality.

腹部からふくらはぎにかけての動脈系の血管造影では異常は見られなかった。

Lesson

Musculoskeletal System　筋骨格系

■ **bone**　骨
- skull (= cranium)　頭蓋骨
  - parietal bone　頭頂骨(とうちょうこつ)
  - frontal bone　前頭骨
  - occipital bone　後頭骨
  - temporal bone　側頭骨
- cheek bone
  - (= zygomatic bone)　頬骨
- upper jaw bone (= maxilla)　上顎骨
- jaw bone (= mandible)　下顎骨
- nasal bone　鼻骨
- backbone (= vertebral
  - column; spine)　脊柱，背骨(背骨全体)
- vertebra (*pl.* vertebrae)　椎骨(ついこつ)
  - cervical vertebrae　頚椎

Further Study
形容詞形も覚えよう！

osseous: 骨の

cranial: 頭蓋の，脳の

spinal: 脊髄の，脊柱の，脊椎の

thoracic vertebrae	胸椎	
lumbar vertebrae	腰椎	
sacral vertebrae	仙椎	
coccygeal vertebrae	尾椎	

intervertebral disk　　椎間〔円〕板
pelvis　　骨盤

Further Study
形容詞形も覚えよう！

pelvic: 骨盤の

 hip bone (= coxal bone)　　寛骨
 sacral bone　　仙骨
 tail bone (= coccygeal bone)　　尾骨
 hip joint　　股関節
collar bone (= clavicle)　　鎖骨
shoulder blade (= scapula)　　肩甲骨
rib (= costa)　　肋骨
breastbone (= sternum)　　胸骨
arm bone (= humerus)　　上腕骨
radius　　橈骨（とうこつ）
ulna　　尺骨
thigh bone (= femur)　　大腿骨
kneecap (= patella)　　膝蓋骨（しつがいこつ）
shin bone (= tibia)　　脛骨（けいこつ）
calf bone (= fibula)　　腓骨（ひこつ）

cartilage　　軟骨

■ **muscle**　　筋肉

muscular: 筋肉の；筋骨たくましい

 smooth muscle　　平滑筋
 skeletal muscle　　骨格筋
 tendon　　腱
 joint (= articulation)　　関節
 ligament　　靭帯（じんたい）

Exercise

● 文章の中で身体の部位名を覚えよう。

太字の日本語に相当する英語を記入し，英文を完成しなさい。

1) _____ is the strong, flexible substance around our joints and in our nose.
   軟骨は関節の周りや鼻の中にある強くて弾力性のある物質である。

2) The _____ in the human body consists of 33 vertebrae.
   人間の**脊柱**は33個の椎骨からできている。

3) The _____ _____ is the ball-and-socket joint connecting the femur and the hipbone.
   股関節は大腿骨と寛骨をつなぐ，電球とソケットのような関節である。

4) A _____ is a tough band of tissue that serves to connect the articular extremities of two bones.
   靭帯とは，骨の関節部分の先端をつなぐ丈夫な結合組織の束のことである。

5) The man over there is the patient with a fractured _____ .
   あそこの男性は，**大腿骨**を骨折した患者だ。

6) There is a crack in the patient's left _____ .
   患者の**橈骨**(とうこつ)にひびが入っている。

Lesson

Blood & Immune System　血液・免疫系

Further Study
形容詞形も覚えよう！

- **heart**　心臓　　　　　　　　　　　　　　　cardiac: 心臓の
  - right atrium　右心房　　　　　　　　　　　atrial: 心房の
  - left atrium　左心房
  - right ventricle　右心室　　　　　　　　　　ventricular: 心室の
  - left ventricle　左心室
  - myocardium (*pl.* myocardia)　心筋　　　　myocardial: 心筋の
  - valve　弁　　　　　　　　　　　　　　　　valvular: 弁の

- **blood vessels**　血管
  - artery　動脈　　　　　　　　　　　　　　　arterial: 動脈の
  - vein　静脈　　　　　　　　　　　　　　　　venous: 静脈の
  - aorta　大動脈　　　　　　　　　　　　　　aortic: 大動脈の
  - superior vena cava　上大静脈
  - inferior vena cava　下大静脈
  - pulmonary artery　肺動脈
  - pulmonary vein　肺静脈
  - coronary artery　冠状動脈
  - carotid artery　頸動脈
  - hepatic portal vein　門脈
  - 〔blood〕capillary　毛細〔血〕管

- **blood**　血液
  - red blood cell
    (= erythrocyte)　赤血球
  - white blood cell
    (= leukocyte)　白血球
  - platelet (= thrombocyte)　血小板
  - plasma　血漿(けっしょう)　　　　　　　　　plasmatic: 血漿の

serum	血清	
monocyte	単〔核〕球	
eosinophilic leukocyte		
（= acidophilic leukocyte)	好酸球	
neutrophil	好中球	
basophil	好塩基球	
phagocyte	食細胞	
macrophage	マクロファージ	

Further Study
形容詞形も覚えよう！

serous: 血清の

■ **lymph**　　　　　　　　リンパ

lymphatic vessels	リンパ管
lymphocyte	リンパ球
B cell (= B lymphocyte)	B 細胞
T cell (= T lymphocyte)	T 細胞
lymph node	リンパ節

spleen (= lien)	脾臓	splenic: 脾臓の
thymus	胸腺	thymic: 胸腺の
bone marrow	骨髄	

Exercise

● 文章の中で身体の部位名を覚えよう。

　太字の日本語に相当する英語を記入し，英文を完成しなさい。

1) The heart is a muscle divided into four chambers known as the right ＿＿＿＿＿ , the right ventricle, the left ＿＿＿＿＿ , and the left ventricle.
   心臓は右**心房**，右心室，左**心房**，左心室として知られる4つの部屋に分かれている筋肉である。

2) The veins from the arms, from the upper trunk and the head and neck, drain into the ＿＿＿＿＿ ＿＿＿＿＿

_____ and on into the right atrium.

腕，上半身や頭部からの静脈は<u>上大静脈</u>を通って右心房へと流れ込む。

4) Blood is made up of millions of red and white blood cells floating in _____ .

血液は<u>血漿</u>の中を浮かんでいる何百万もの赤血球，白血球からできている。

5) Cells within the lymph nodes such as _____ and microphage engulf cellular debris and bacteria and help produce antibodies.

リンパ節中の<u>マクロファージ</u>やミクロファージは細胞の断片やバクテリアを貪食し，抗体をつくりだすのを助ける。

Lesson

Respiratory System	**呼吸器系**
nose	鼻
nostril	鼻孔
nasal cavity	鼻腔
paranasal sinus	副鼻腔
nasopharynx	鼻咽頭
uvula	口蓋垂
throat	喉
pharynx	咽頭
pharyngeal tonsil	咽頭扁桃
epiglottis	喉頭蓋
larynx (= voice box)	喉頭
trachea (= windpipe)	気管
vocal cord (= vocal folds)	声帯
glottis	声門

Further Study
形容詞形も覚えよう！

nasal: 鼻の

pharyngeal: 咽頭の

laryngeal: 喉頭の
tracheal: 気管の

bronchus (*pl.* bronchi; 　= bronchial tube)	気管支	
bronchiole	細気管支（気管支が6回以上 　　　　分岐して以後の細径のもの）	
lung	肺	
alveolus	肺胞	
pleura (*pl.* pleurae)	胸膜，肋膜	
diaphragm	横隔膜（おうかくまく）	

Further Study
形容詞形も覚えよう！

bronchial: 気管支の

pulmonary: 肺の

alveolar: 肺胞の

pleural: 胸膜の

diaphragmatic: 横隔膜の

Exercise

● 文章の中で身体の部位名を覚えよう。

太字の日本語に相当する英語を記入し，英文を完成しなさい。

1) The inspired air passes from the _____ _____ by way of the nasopharynx and pharynx to the larynx.
   呼吸で吸い込まれた空気は，<u>鼻腔</u>から鼻咽頭と咽頭を通って喉頭へと行く。

2) The _____ divides into two main branches called the primary bronchi.
   <u>気管</u>は主気管支と呼ばれる2つの主な枝に分かれる。

3) The _____ is a serous membrane that surrounds the outer covering of each lung.
   <u>胸膜</u>は両肺それぞれの外表面を覆う漿液性の粘膜である。

4) The _____ is the muscle which separates the thoracic cavity (lungs and heart) from the abdominal cavity.
   <u>横隔膜</u>は胸郭（肺と心臓）と腹腔を分ける筋肉である。

Lesson

Digestive System　　消化器系

- **oral cavity**　　口腔

    mouth　　口

    lip　　唇

    tongue (= lingua; glossa)　　舌　　　　　　　　　　　lingual; glossal: 舌の

    　taste bud　　味蕾

    tooth　　歯

    　gum (= gingiva)　　歯肉，歯茎(はぐき)　　　　　　gingival: 歯肉の

    　incisor　　切歯(せっし)

    　canine (【俗】eyetooth)　　犬歯(けんし)

    　molar　　大臼歯(だいきゅうし)

    　wisdom tooth　　親知らず

    　crown　　歯冠

    　enamel　　エナメル質

    　dentin　　象牙質

    　dental pulp　　歯髄

    　root　　歯根

    　permanent tooth

    　　(【俗】adult tooth)　　永久歯

    　deciduous tooth

    　　(【俗】baby tooth)　　乳歯

    pharynx　　咽頭　　　　　　　　　　　　　　　　　　pharyngeal: 咽頭の

    tonsil　　扁桃　　　　　　　　　　　　　　　　　　　tonsillar: 扁桃の

    esophagus　　食道　　　　　　　　　　　　　　　　　esophageal: 食道の

- **stomach**　　胃　　　　　　　　　　　　　　　　　　　gastric: 胃の

    cardia　　噴門　　　　　　　　　　　　　　　　　　　cardiac: 噴門の；心臓の

    pylorus　　幽門　　　　　　　　　　　　　　　　　　　pyloric: 幽門の

Further Study
形容詞形も覚えよう！

- **small intestine ([俗] small bowel)　　小腸**

duodenum	十二指腸	duodenal: 十二指腸の
jejunum	空腸	jejunal: 空腸の
ileum	回腸	ileal; ileac: 回腸の

- **large intestine ([俗] large bowel; colon)　　大腸**

colon	結腸	colonic: 結腸の
ascending colon	上行結腸	
transverse colon	横行結腸	
descending colon	下行結腸	
sigmoid colon	S状結腸	
cecum	盲腸	cecal: 盲腸の
appendix	虫垂	
rectum	直腸	rectal: 直腸の
anus	肛門	anal: 肛門の

liver	肝臓	hepatic: 肝臓の
gallbladder	胆嚢(たんのう)	
pancreas	膵臓(すいぞう)	pancreatic: 膵臓の
villus (*pl.* villi)	絨毛	

Exercise

● 文章の中で身体の部位名を覚えよう。

太字の日本語に相当する英語を記入し，英文を完成しなさい。

1) The oral cavity is the entrance to the long tubular _____ system, which consists of the lips, mouth, pharynx, esophagus, stomach, small and large intestine, rectum, and anus.

   口腔は，唇，口，咽頭，食道，胃，小腸，大腸，直腸，そして肛門から成る長い<u>消化管</u>の入り口である。

2) The _____ is a small rounded mass of lymphoid tissue.
   扁桃は小さく丸い，リンパ組織の塊である。

3) The _____ is a muscular tube 25 cm in length that conveys food from the pharynx to the stomach.
   食道は食物を咽頭から胃へと運ぶ長さ 25 cm の筋肉の管である。

4) When the food enters the _____ , it is mixed with the gastric juice by the action of the strong muscular _____ _____ _____ _____ .
   食物は胃に入ると，胃壁の強力な筋肉の動きにより胃液と混ぜ合わされる。

5) The lining of the small intestine is covered with thousands of very small projections called _____ .
   小腸の内壁は絨毛と呼ばれる何千もの非常に小さな突起で覆われている。

6) _____ is the part of the large intestine extending from the cecum to the rectum.
   結腸は盲腸から直腸まで伸びる大腸の部分である。

7) The functions of the _____ include storage and filtration of blood, secretion of bile, conversion of sugars into glycogen, and many other metabolic activities.
   肝臓の機能には，血液の貯蔵や濾過（ろか），胆汁の分泌，ブドウ糖のグリコーゲンへの転化，そして他の多くの代謝活動などがある。

8) The _____ is a pear-shaped, hollow organ closely attached to the posterior surface of the liver and containing bile.
   胆嚢は，肝臓の後ろ側の表面に密着している梨状の臓器で胆汁を貯蔵している。

9) The _____ is a large, elongated, racemose gland situated transversely behind the stomach, between the spleen and duodenum.

   膵臓は胃の後ろ側，脾臓と十二指腸の間に位置する，大きく長く伸びた，蔓(つる)状の腺である。

Lesson

Urinary System	泌尿器系
kidney	腎臓
renal pelvis	腎盂
ureter	尿管
urinary bladder	膀胱(ぼうこう)
urethra	尿道
urine	尿

Further Study
形容詞形も覚えよう！

renal: 腎臓の

ureteral; ureteric: 尿管の

urethral: 尿道の

uric; urinary: 尿の

Exercise

●文章の中で身体の部位名を覚えよう。

太字の日本語に相当する英語を記入し，英文を完成しなさい。

1) The _____ take waste matter from your blood and send it out of your body as urine.

   <u>腎臓</u>は血液中の老廃物を取り除き，それを尿として体外に送り出す。

2) The _____ receives urine from the kidneys by way of the ureters and discharges it to the urethra.

   尿は腎臓から尿管を通って<u>膀胱</u>へ入り，そこから尿道へと排泄される。

Lesson

Endocrine System　　内分泌系

hypothalamus	視床下部
pituitary gland	下垂体
pineal gland	松果体(しょうかたい)
thyroid gland	甲状腺
parathyroid gland	上皮小体，副甲状腺
adrenal gland	副腎(ふくじん)
medulla of suprarenal gland	副腎髄質
adrenal cortex	副腎皮質
pancreas	膵臓(すいぞう)
Langerhans islands	ランゲルハンス島

Further Study
形容詞形も覚えよう！

hypothalamic: 視床下部の

Exercise

● 文章の中で身体の部位名を覚えよう。

太字の日本語に相当する英語を記入し，英文を完成しなさい。

1) Women have larger and more easily palpable _____ _____ than men.

   女性の**甲状腺**は男性よりも大きくて触診しやすい。

2) _____ produces insulin and substances that help your body digest food.

   膵臓はインスリンと食物の消化を助ける物質をつくっている。

Lesson

Reproductive System (Genital System) 生殖器系

■ **male genital organs**　　男性生殖器

testis (*pl.* testes; = testicle)	精巣(せいそう)，睾丸
deferent duct (= ductus deferens)	精管
seminal vesicles	精囊(せいのう)
sperm (= spermatozoon)	精子
scrotum	陰囊(いんのう)
prostate〔gland〕	前立腺
penis	陰茎(いんけい)

Further Study　形容詞形も覚えよう！

testicular: 精巣の

scrotal: 陰囊の
prostatic: 前立腺の

Exercise

● 文章の中で身体の部位名を覚えよう。

太字の日本語に相当する英語を記入し，英文を完成しなさい。

1) The head of a mature _____ contains a nucleus with all of the genetic traits a father can transmit to his offspring.

　成熟した**精子**の頭部は，父親が子孫に伝えうるすべての遺伝的特徴を伝える核をもっている。

2) Testosterone is secreted by the _____ .

　テストステロンは**精巣**から分泌される。

Lesson

■ **female genital organs**　　女性生殖器

ovary	卵巣
ovarian follicle	卵胞
oocyte	卵母細胞

ovarian: 卵巣の

ovum	卵子	oval: 卵子の；卵形の
uterine tube (= fallopian tube)	卵管	
uterus (= womb)	子宮	uterine: 子宮の
fundus of uterus	子宮底	
(= fundus uteri)	子宮頸	
cervix of uterus		
(= cervix uteri)	子宮口	
orifice of uterus		
(= ostium uteri)		
vagina	腟	vaginal: 腟の
perineum	会陰	perineal: 会陰の
clitoris	陰核	clitoridean: 陰核の
umbilical cord	臍帯(さいたい)	
placenta	胎盤	placental: 胎盤の
embryo	胚(発育初期の生物)；胎芽	embryonic: 胚の
fetus	胎児	fetal: 胎児の
mammary gland	乳腺	

Further Study
形容詞形も覚えよう！

＊ヒトでは，受胎から8週の終わりまでを embryo（胎芽），妊娠第8週の終わりから出生時までを fetus（胎児）といいます。

Exercise

● 文章の中で身体の部位名を覚えよう。

太字の日本語に相当する英語を記入し，英文を完成しなさい。

1) The _____ develops and matures ova and discharges them into the pelvic cavity.

   卵巣は卵子を発達・成熟させ，骨盤腔に排出する。

2) The _____ is composed of an endometrium and a myometrium.

   子宮は子宮内膜と子宮筋で構成されている。

3) The _____ is the mass of veins and tissue which the fetus is attached to inside the womb of a pregnant woman.

<u>胎盤</u>は妊婦の子宮内にある血管と組織の塊で，胎児がそこにつながっている。

Lesson

Nervous System 神経系

■ **brain**	脳	
cerebrum	大脳	cerebral: 大脳の
cerebral cortex	大脳皮質	
frontal lobe	前頭葉	lobar: 葉の
parietal lobe	頭頂葉	
occipital lobe	後頭葉	
temporal lobe	側頭葉	
hippocampus	海馬	hippocampal: 海馬の
basal ganglia	大脳基底核	
cerebellum	小脳	cerebellar: 小脳の
brainstem	脳幹	
diencephalon (*pl.* diencephala)	間脳	
thalamus	視床	
hypothalamus	視床下部	hypothalamic: 視床下部の
medulla oblongata	延髄	
midbrain	中脳	
pons	橋	
spinal cord	脊髄	
meninx (*pl.* meninges)	髄膜	meningeal: 髄膜の
dura mater	硬膜	
pia mater	軟膜	
arachnoid membrane	くも膜	

Further Study 形容詞形も覚えよう！

- **central nervous system**　　中枢神経系
  - cranial nerves　　脳神経
  - spinal nerves　　脊髄神経
  - peripheral nerves　　末梢神経
  - autonomic nerves　　自律神経
  - sympathetic nerves　　交感神経
  - parasympathetic nerves　　副交感神経

  - neuron　　ニューロン，神経単位
  - dendrites　　樹状突起
  - cell body　　細胞体
  - synapse　　シナプス，接合〔部〕
  - axon　　軸索
  - myelin〔sheath〕　　ミエリン〔鞘〕；髄鞘

Further Study
形容詞形も覚えよう！

nervous: 神経の；神経質な

neural: 神経の

neuronal: ニューロンの

dendritic: 樹状突起の

cellular: 細胞の

synaptic: シナプスの

axonal: 軸索の

myelinic: ミエリンの

Exercise

● 文章の中で身体の部位名を覚えよう。

太字の日本語に相当する英語を記入し，英文を完成しなさい。

1) The _____ , which forms the base of the brain, coordinates all movement and helps maintain the body upright in space.

   脳の底部にある**小脳**は，すべての動きを調整し，空間で体が直立しつづけることを助ける。

2) The _____ connects the cerebral hemispheres of the brain with the spinal cord.

   脳幹は，脳の上部と脊髄とをつなげている。

3) The _____ _____ is a thick cord of nerves inside your spine which connects your brain to nerves in all parts of your body.

   脊髄は脊椎の中の神経の太い束で，脳と全身の神経を結

4) The _____ _____ of the brain has two layers, both consisting of connective tissue with elongated fibroblasts.

脳の**硬膜**は，結合組織と長く伸びた線維芽細胞から成る2層構造になっている。

5) The _____ consists of cell bodies and their axons, single long fibers that conduct impulses to other parts of the nervous system.

ニューロンは，細胞体と，神経の活動電位を他の神経系に伝える長い線維である軸索とから成っている。

6) The _____ _____ _____ consists of the brain and the spinal cord, and the _____ consists of the 12 pairs of cranial nerves and the autonomic nervous system.

中枢神経系は脳と脊髄から成り，**末梢神経系**は12対の脳神経と，脊髄神経および自律神経系から成っている。

COLUMN

杉田玄白と前野良沢

　日本の医学史をひもとくと，医師たちが外国語習得に悪戦苦闘したことがよくわかります。江戸時代の鎖国下で解剖学書『ターヘル・アナトミア』を杉田玄白たちが3年以上の歳月をかけて翻訳して『解体新書』として刊行した際の並外れた苦労話は，つとに有名です（ドイツ人クルムスによる原著をオランダ語に翻訳したもの）。この翻訳は前野良沢の貢献なしには完成しなかったのですが，なぜか訳者名から良沢の名は削除されています。それは刊行を急ぐ玄白に対して，良沢は訳がまだ不完全であるとして良心から自分の名前を公にすることを辞退したためと考えられています。その後，玄白はオランダ語の研究をやめ，蘭方医として名声と富を手に入れ，一方，学究肌の良沢は，貧しい生活の中でオランダ語研究を続け，医学ばかりでなく，天文学・暦学・地理などの訳書を残しました。

Lesson

Sensory Organs　　　　感覚器官

■ **visual organ**　　　　視覚器官

eye	目
eyeball	眼球
sclera	強膜
conjunctiva	結膜
cornea	角膜
iris	虹彩
pupil	瞳孔
ciliary body	毛様体
lens	水晶体
vitreous body	硝子体
(= hyaloid body)	
retina	網膜
optic nerve	視神経
macula of retina	黄斑
central retinal fovea	中心窩
lacrimal gland	涙腺
(= lachrymal gland)	

Further Study
形容詞形も覚えよう！

scleral: 強膜の

conjunctival: 結膜の

corneal: 角膜の

pupillary: 瞳孔の

lenticular: 水晶体の，レンズ形の

retinal: 網膜の

macular: 黄斑の

Exercise

● 文章の中で身体の部位名を覚えよう。

太字の日本語に相当する英語を記入し，英文を完成しなさい。

1) The _____ is transparent, permitting the rays of light to enter.

　光が入っていくように，**角膜**は透明である。

2) The _____ contains the receptors for light and the complex neural networks which send impulses of the

visual information through the optic nerve to the brain.
網膜は光の受容体と，視覚情報のインパルスを視神経を通して脳に送る複雑な神経ネットワークとをもっている。

Lesson

■ **auditory organ**	聴覚器官
outer ear (= auris externa)	外耳
auricle	耳介
earlobe	耳たぶ
external〔ear〕canal	外耳道
(= external auditory meatus)	
middle ear (= auris media)	中耳
eardrum	
(= tympanic membrane)	鼓膜
tympanic cavity	鼓室
ear bones (= auditory ossicles)	耳小骨
malleus	ツチ骨
incus	キヌタ骨
stapes	アブミ骨
auditory tube	耳管
inner ear (= auris interna)	内耳
oval window	前庭窓
semicircular duct	三半規管
cochlear duct	蝸牛管

Further Study
形容詞形も覚えよう！

auricular: 耳介の；心耳の

Exercise

● 文章の中で身体の部位名を覚えよう。

太字の日本語に相当する英語を記入し，英文を完成しなさい。

1) The middle ear comprises the tympanic cavity, the

_____ _____ , its contents, the auditory tube, and the tympanic membrane.

中耳は，鼓室とその中にある**耳小骨**，耳管，そして鼓膜から成っている。

2) The _____ _____ is shaped like a very flat cone with its apex directed medially.

鼓膜は先端が内側に向いている非常に平らな円錐形をしている。

Lesson

Skin 皮膚

epidermis (*pl.* epidermides)	表皮
dermis	真皮
subcutaneous tissue	皮下組織
pore	毛穴
hair follicle	毛包
duct of sweat gland	汗腺
sebaceous glands	〔皮〕脂腺
nail	爪
nail plate	爪板
lunula (*pl.* lunulae)	半月

Further Study
形容詞形も覚えよう！

cutaneous: 皮膚の

epidermal: 表皮の，上皮性の

dermal: 真皮の，皮膚の

Exercise

● 文章の中で身体の部位名を覚えよう。

太字の日本語に相当する英語を記入し，英文を完成しなさい。

1) _____ protect the distal ends of the fingers and toes.

爪は手指や足指の先を保護する。

2) The _____ depends on the underlying dermis for

its nutrition.

表皮はその下にある真皮から栄養を得ている。

3) _____ _____ produce a fatty substance that is secreted onto the skin surface through the hair follicles.

皮脂腺は，脂肪分を毛包を通して皮膚表面に分泌する。

Lesson

Miscellaneous　　その他

body fluid	体液
tissue fluid	組織液
cerebrospinal fluid	髄液
mucus	粘液
saliva	唾液
bile	胆汁
gastric juice	胃液
pancreatic juice	膵液
semen	精液
pus	膿（のう）
sputum (= phlegm)	痰（たん）
sweat	汗
stool (= feces)	大便
urine	尿
membrane	膜
mucosa	粘膜
dandruff	ふけ
earwax	耳垢
eye matter; eye discharge (= ophthalmorrhea)	目やに
amniotic fluid	羊水

Further Study
形容詞形も覚えよう！

mucous: 粘液の

salivary: 唾液の

seminal: 精液の

uric; urinary: 尿の

membranous: 膜の，膜状の

mucosal: 粘膜の

Part 3
Listening to Medical News

Part 3: Listening to Medical News

Chapter 6 Listening to Medical News (1)

POINT ☞ 一般向けニュース番組で取り上げられた医療トピックを聴き，そこで使われている表現を学ぼう。

Listening

Silent Killer

Before Listening 下記の医学用語は英語で何というでしょうか？ 本文中から探してみましょう。

1. 糖尿病　　　＿＿＿＿＿＿＿
2. 渇水感　　　＿＿＿＿＿＿＿
3. 診断する　　＿＿＿＿＿＿＿
4. 排尿　　　　＿＿＿＿＿＿＿
5. 合併症　　　＿＿＿＿＿＿＿
6. 血管　　　　＿＿＿＿＿＿＿
7. 心臓病　　　＿＿＿＿＿＿＿
8. 腎臓　　　　＿＿＿＿＿＿＿

First Listening 下線部を聴き取り，記入してみましょう。

Elizabeth Vargas: We're going to take "A Closer Look" tonight at a silent killer, diabetes. There is a study in tomorrow's *New England Journal of Medicine* that says losing weight and exercising can dramatically reduce the risk of adults developing diabetes.

A regimen that could easily help so many people. 16 million Americans have diabetes but a startling number of them, about a third, do not know it until the damage is already done. Here's ABC's John McKenzie.

John McKenzie: Ask Americans a basic question about their health and many think they know the answer. Do you have (1) _____ ?

Lady: No.

John McKenzie: How do you know?

Lady: Uh ... I'm assuming.

John McKenzie: Excuse me. Do you have (1) _____ ?

Gentleman: No, I don't.

John McKenzie: How do you know?

Gentleman: Uh ... I don't know.

John McKenzie: Can I ask you a quick question? Do you have (1) _____ ?

Another Lady: Nope.

John McKenzie: How do you know?

Another Lady: How do I know ... I don't have any (2) _____ .

Dr. Alan Moses: The classic (2) _____ of (1) _____ are increased (3) _____ , increased (4) _____ and general lack of energy or weakness. Unfortunately, many people have (1) _____ and they don't know it because they don't have those (2) _____ .

John McKenzie: And they (5) _____ _____ _____ _____ for years.

Dr. David Nathan: During that time the (1) _____ is causing its damage, causing its mischief with

regimen: 養生法，療法

nope (= no; ⇔ yep)

(6) _____ _____ in the eyes and the (7) _____ and maybe even causing and leading to heart disease.

John McKenzie: Adults develop (1) _____ when their bodies (8) _____ _____ _____ _____ . So doctors diagnose the disease by looking for high levels of sugar or glucose in the blood. The American Diabetes Association says everyone 45 and older should have this test at least every three years. And because the test can detect levels even slightly higher than normal, it can identify a problem before it turns into diabetes. That's important because the study in tomorrow's *New England Journal of Medicine* shows that people with (9) _____ _____ _____ _____ _____ _____ in their blood can avoid developing diabetes by simple changes in their lifestyle. Specifically, losing at least 7% of body weight and increasing physical activity, usually brisk walking thirty minutes a day, was enough to reduce the risk of developing diabetes by 58%.

Dr. David Nathan: We need not wait for them to get (1) _____ and then the (10) _____ of (1)_____ . We can do something about it earlier.

John McKenzie: A simple but often overlooked blood test. That's critical in identifying those at risk for diabetes and those who already have it.

John McKenzie, ABC News, New York.

Silent Killer (ABC News, February 6, 2002)
Reprinted with permission.

diagnose: 診断する

brisk: 活発な，きびきびした

Chapter 6　Medical News (1)

Second Listening　本文の内容と一致するものにはT，一致しないものにはFを付けてみましょう。

1. Few people with diabetes know its symptoms.
   糖尿病の病識がある人は少ない。　　　　　_____

2. The symptoms of diabetes are thirst, increased urination and general lack of energy.
   糖尿病の症状は，のどの渇き，頻尿，全身の倦怠感などである。　　　　　_____

3. Even slightly higher than normal levels of sugar in the blood does not identify a problem.
   血糖値が少々高くても，血液検査で問題になることはない。　　　　　_____

4. A study shows that people with higher than normal levels of sugar in the blood can avoid developing diabetes by changing their lifestyle.
   血糖値が高くても生活習慣を変えることで，糖尿病を予防できるとする研究がある。　　　　　_____

63

Listening

Autism: Early Signs

Before Listening 下記の医学用語は英語で何というでしょうか？ 本文中から探してみましょう。

1. 自閉症　　　　＿＿＿＿＿＿＿
2. 発達障害　　　＿＿＿＿＿＿＿
3. 早期診断　　　＿＿＿＿＿＿＿
4. 出生　　　　　＿＿＿＿＿＿＿
5. 小児科医　　　＿＿＿＿＿＿＿

First Listening 下線部を聴き取り，記入してみましょう。

Peter Jennings: We're going to take a closer look tonight at what we are told is a major advance in the fight against autism. Autism is a developmental disorder of childhood. It is characterized by (1) ＿＿＿＿＿＿ ＿＿＿＿ ＿＿＿＿ ＿＿＿＿ ＿＿＿＿ . It is heartbreaking for parents. The government says that about one in every 250 children is diagnosed with autism. This report tonight is about early diagnosis, which could make a huge difference. Here's ABC's John McKenzie.

John McKenzie: Loren Anderson is a year old. Her parents are worried because she is not developing normally and they think she may have autism.

Shani Anderson, Mother: Hitting her head on people in an aggressive fashion, hitting her head on hard objects repeatedly, she just learned to crawl on all fours.

> it is characterized by ...:
> …を特徴とする

Chapter 6   Medical News (1)

John McKenzie: (2) _____ _____ _____ _____ _____ until children are three years old or later when most of the damage to the developing brain may have already been done. But in studies at the Kennedy Krieger Institute in Baltimore, researchers are following children from birth and can now spot troubling signs of autism at six months of age and actually (3) _____ _____ _____ in children as young as fourteen months.

Prof. Rebecca Landa, Kennedy Krieger Institute: One of the things that's coming out of the research today is that you cannot look at just one behavior or one domain of development. You have to look across developmental domains.

John McKenzie: According to the new research, at six months of age the possible signs of autism include babies who do not (4) _____ , _____ _____ _____ _____ _____ with people. (Typically developing babies are engaged.) As the child grows, researchers look for other alarming patterns. At one year the possible signs include toddlers who do not gesture such as (5) _____ and _____ or who do not _____ _____ or _____ with people. While autism can now be diagnosed in younger children, researchers say many pediatricians are not looking for signs early enough and ordering the necessary testing. (6) _____ _____ _____ _____ can lead to _____ _____ . And the study showed the earlier the therapy begins, the less impact autism has on the brain.

Prof. Rebecca Landa: To the point where we can really

toddler: よちよち歩く人，歩きはじめの子供

help children engage socially, speed along their development of language, help them become aware of peers.

John McKenzie: In short, allowing them to lead more normal lives.

John McKenzie, ABC News, New York.

Autism: Early Signs (ABC News, April 22, 2004)
Reprinted with permission.

Second Listening　本文の内容と一致するものには **T**，一致しないものには **F** を付けてみましょう。

1. Autistic children cannot go out of their room.
   自閉症の子どもは自分の部屋から出ることができない。
   ＿＿＿

2. Ms. Anderson is very concerned about her daughter because she thinks the child may have autism.
   アンダーソンさんは娘が自閉症かも知れないので，娘のことを心配している。
   ＿＿＿

3. Children with autism tend to smile, babble or make eye contact with people.
   自閉症の子どもは，笑ったり，片言を言ったり，人とアイコンタクトをしがちである。
   ＿＿＿

4. Early testing and diagnosis is the key to the treatment of autism.
   早期の検査と診断が自閉症の治療には大切だ。　＿＿＿

COLUMN

医学英語にはなぜギリシャ語源とラテン語源が多いのか？　②ラテン語を仲介したフランス語

　現在のイングランド人の祖先は，ヨーロッパ北方民族であったアングロ人とサクソン人です。

　ブリテン島には1世紀頃からローマ帝国が侵攻し，現在のイングランドに相当する地域を支配しました。そして先住民であったケルト人が逃れた先が，現在のスコットランドやウェールズに相当する地域です。

　ローマ帝国が崩壊すると，イングランド各地でも争乱が起こり，その戦いの傭兵としてアングロ人とサクソン人が呼ばれたのですが，やがてその彼らが数を増し，イングランドの実権を握ることになったのです。

　そのため言語もアングロ-サクソン人の言語である低地ゲルマン語が使用され，それが独自の発達を遂げて現在の英語が成立したのです。古期英語とよばれる時代（450～1100）には，当時は高度な文明であったローマ帝国の言語であるラテン語の影響が続きました。例えばcancer, paralysis, plasterのような医学英語は，この時代にラテン語から英語に借入されています。

　またラテン語の英語への影響に触れるとき，イングランドへの侵略者の言語であるフランス語を無視することはできません。フランス語は言語的にラテン語族であり，歴史的にもローマ帝国の影響を強く受けています。そのフランス語が，1066年のノルマンディー侯ウィリアムのイングランド征服以来約200年間，イングランド上層階級の共通言語となりましたが，一般庶民は英語を使っていました。

　その後，フランスとの百年戦争（1337～1453）の間にイングランド人は上層階級もフランス語を排して英語を使うようになりましたが，庶民のことばだった英語を使って政治や経済，文化，学問などを早急にイングランド人の言語として定着させるために，当時の英語になかった語彙をラテン語から取り込んだのです。

　またその後16世紀のルネサンス時代には，印刷機の普及によってギリシャ語やラテン語で書かれた大量の古典が英語に翻訳されましたが，このときも英語にない語彙を補うためにギリシャ語とラテン語が大量に英語に流入しました。

　同様の現象が医学分野の用語にも起こり，ギリシャ語やラテン語そのもの，あるいはフランス語が同化した英語が大きな割合を占めているというわけです。

　またこのような歴史的背景から，英語には他の言語を柔軟に取り入れる下地がつくられました。現在でも最新の医学研究の現場では，新しい専門用語がギリシャ語やラテン語をもとにつくられ続けています。

Part 3: Listening to Medical News

Chapter 7 Listening to Medical News (2)

POINT ☞ 一般向けニュース番組で取り上げられた医療トピックを聴き，そこで使われている表現を学ぼう。

Listening

Coping with SARS in the U.S.

Before Listening 下記の医学用語は英語で何というでしょうか？本文中から探してみましょう。

1. 新型肺炎　　　　　　　　＿＿＿＿＿＿
2. 重症急性呼吸器症候群　　＿＿＿＿＿＿
3. 回復する　　　　　　　　＿＿＿＿＿＿
4. 〔容態が〕悪化する　　　＿＿＿＿＿＿
5. 罹患する　　　　　　　　＿＿＿＿＿＿
6. 〔感染症を〕封じ込める　＿＿＿＿＿＿

First Listening 下線部を聴き取り，記入してみましょう。

Susan Dentzer: Kurk Lew and his 11-year-old daughter Amanda are U.S. citizens from Virginia. They still (1) ＿＿＿＿ ＿＿＿＿ ＿＿＿＿ ＿＿＿＿ to Lew's native China. In January they returned there for a visit, taking along Lew's 72-year-old aunt. It was the aunt's first visit to her native land in 20 years.

Kurk Lew: She was very, very healthy, and she walked,

she walked ... she visited a lot of places, you know, so she was never tired. She was so excited because she had seen so many new things there, you know, since the last time she went back there.

Susan Dentzer: But the joyful homecoming soured when Lew's aunt became ill in the midst of the trip.

Amanda Lew: Somewhere along the way she got a flu-like ... flu-like symptoms. And then when she got back to her hometown, she was tired, and she ate barely anything.

Susan Dentzer: The aunt's condition continued to deteriorate once she was home in Virginia. Lew telephoned his own father back in China.

deteriorate: 悪化する

Kurk Lew: My father said, "You may want to take some precautions, you know, because there was an epidemic they called atypical pneumonia going on, and you may want to watch her, you know, more carefully."

precaution: 用心，注意

epidemic: 流行病の発生

atypical: 非定型の，異型の

Susan Dentzer: Days later, the aunt was (2) _____ _____ _____ to this Virginia hospital, where she spent ten difficult days. She's now fully recovered, but did not want to be interviewed on camera. Public health experts believe her illness was America's first probable case of the disease now known as SARS.

public health: 公衆衛生

SARS (= Severe Acute Respiratory Syndrome): 重症急性呼吸器症候群，新型肺炎

Kurk Lew: You want to take a quick trip and then all of a sudden you catch this type of thing and then it's ... then you almost ... I would say almost die, you know. Because, you know, she feels very, very lucky.

Susan Dentzer: Aside from luck, Lew's aunt (3) _____ _____ _____ _____ _____ from _____ _____ _____ and the _____

_____ _____ .

Dr. Julie Gerberding: This is one of the ways that we track the global epidemic.

Susan Dentzer: Dr. Julie Gerberding, who directs the U.S. Centers for Disease Control and Prevention in Atlanta, says that's one reason the U.S. has so far experienced many fewer SARS cases than other countries.

Dr. Julie Gerberding: We've taken very broad steps to contain the spread once we have a suspicious case, and our public health officials have done an (4) _____ _____ _____ _____ _____ _____ _____ so that we have done everything we can to isolate people as early as possible.

case: 症例

Global disease experts say the SARS virus first appeared in China last fall, in the southern province of Guangdong. From Guangdong, a few key individuals inadvertently transmitted the virus to many more people in other parts of China and the rest of the world.

virus: ウイルス
Guangdong: 広東
inadvertently: 不注意に

Public health experts have dubbed them "super-spreaders" or "hypertransmitters." For example, almost all SARS cases in Canada can be traced to a single elderly Chinese immigrant. She apparently contracted the disease in a Hong Kong hotel, and died soon after returning to Toronto. But (5) _____ _____ of her family _____ _____ _____ _____ _____ to health care workers.

immigrant: 移民

Public health experts say they don't know why some people are super-spreaders and they say other factors may explain the phenomenon. But for whatever reason, they say, Kurk Lew's aunt was not one of them. Had she been, (6) _____ _____ _____ ____ _____ _____ _____ .

Coping with SARS in the U.S. (NewsHour, April 29, 2003)
Reprinted with permission.

Second Listening   本文の内容と一致するものには **T**，一致しないものには **F** を付けてみましょう。

1. The symptoms of SARS are similar to those of the flu.
   SARS の症状は，インフルエンザの症状と似ている。 _____

2. The SARS patient was an 11-year-old Chinese-American girl.
   SARS の患者は，11 歳の中国系米国人少女だった。 _____

3. Unfortunately, the first SARS patient in the U.S. died.
   米国での最初の SARS 患者は不幸にも亡くなった。 _____

4. The SARS virus first appeared in the southern province of Guangdong, China.
   SARS は広東省南部で最初に発生したようである。 _____

Listening

Caring for the First SARS Patient in the U.S.

Before Listening　下記の医学用語は英語で何というでしょうか？本文中から探してみましょう。

1. 流行病　　　　＿＿＿＿＿＿＿
2. 抗生物質　　　＿＿＿＿＿＿＿
3. 陰圧式　　　　＿＿＿＿＿＿＿
4. 死亡率　　　　＿＿＿＿＿＿＿
5. 脱水状態の　　＿＿＿＿＿＿＿

First Listening　下線部を聴き取り，記入してみましょう。

Susan Dentzer: Karin Kerby is a nurse at Loudoun General Hospital in Leesburg, Virginia. She was in charge of the emergency room on Monday February 17, when Lew's aunt arrived at the hospital.

Karin Kerby, RN*, Loudoun General Hospital: I was made aware of a woman that they were moving into a room who had a bad pneumonia, and that was what I was told. Mrs ... this woman needed to be in a room, to be (1) ＿＿＿＿ ＿＿＿＿＿ , because she had a ＿＿＿＿＿＿ ＿＿＿＿＿＿ .

Susan Dentzer: For several hours, the aunt lay in a bed in this emergency room. At that point, no (2) ＿＿＿＿＿＿ ＿＿＿＿＿＿ were being taken against ＿＿＿＿＿ ＿＿＿＿＿ ＿＿＿＿＿ ＿＿＿＿＿ . Eventually a worried Lew, having learned that his aunt was at the hospital, telephoned Nurse Kerby there.

emergency room (ER): 救急救命室

*RN (R.N.) = registered nurse
cf. LPN (= licensed practical nurse), LVN (= licensed vocational nurse)

pneumonia: 肺炎

Kurk Lew: And I said, well, my aunt went to China, and there was an epidemic going on there and they called it atypical pneumonia. And I said, you know, there is a possibility that she might have caught it.

Karin Kerby: I had read in the newspaper the week before a little article about a pneumonia that was atypical in China that had a high mortality rate. So I put that knowledge together with what he was telling me, and red flags went off.

Susan Dentzer: The (3) _____ _____ _____ _____ _____ _____ _____ _____ from a plan initially drawn up for responding to _____ _____ _____ _____ . First, they called the local Loudoun County public health department. Dr. David Goodfriend is the director.

Dr. David Goodfriend, Loudoun County Public Health Dept.: Our staff, in consultation with the hospital, made sure that she was put in an appropriate isolation precaution so that no one else in the hospital, no other patients would (4) _____ _____ _____ _____ _____ _____ until we had a chance to work her up and make sure that she couldn't _____ _____ _____ to other people.

Susan Dentzer: That meant putting Lew's aunt into a special room equipped with so-called negative pressure airflow.

Karin Kerby: Someone with a (5) _____ _____ usually can _____ _____ _____ _____ _____ or _____ _____ _____ _____ _____ _____ _____ . So by turning on the ventilation system, it at least began the process of

ventilation: 換気

taking the infection away from the rest of the emergency department.

Susan Dentzer: Kerby and other members of the hospital staff also took other precautions. They (6) _____ _____ _____ , _____ and _____ , or _____ _____ , to enter the _____ _____ .

They then discarded those protective coverings and scrubbed up as they left. All these steps may have helped to prevent hospital workers from becoming sick, as had already begun to happen in Canada.

Dr. Antonio Pastor is an infectious disease specialist who was called in to treat Lew's aunt. He told us that her chest X-rays revealed clouded areas of the lungs.

Dr. Antonio Pastor, Infectious Disease Specialist: We put her on oxygen, we gave her fluids — she was also dehydrated — and put her on a combination of very potent antibiotics, and, you know, she started to respond very quickly.

Susan Dentzer: SARS is viral; why did the antibiotics work?

Dr. Antonio Pastor: It's very possible that she had this viral infection with a superimposed bacterial infection. So her immune system pretty much responded well to the viral infection, the SARS, but then she had this superimposed bacterial infection, and that's why I think the antibiotics were so beneficial for her.

Coping with SARS in the U.S. (NewsHour, April 29, 2003)
Reprinted with permission.

---

infection: 感染

discard: 廃棄する，処分する

scrub: ごしごしこすって洗う

fluid: 体液
dehydrated: 脱水した
antibiotics: 抗生物質

viral infection: ウイルス感染

superimpose: 重ねる，上乗せする

immune system: 免疫系

Chapter 7　Medical News (2)

Second Listening　本文の内容と一致するものには **T**，一致しないものには **F** を付けてみましょう。

1. Nurse Kerby raised a red flag when she saw the patient.
   カービー看護師はその患者さんを見て警鐘を鳴らした。
   _____

2. The emergency room staff were not prepared for possible instances of bioterrorism.
   救急部のスタッフは生物兵器テロの可能性に対して準備をしていなかった。
   _____

3. Lew's aunt was placed on the respirator.
   ルーの叔母さんは人工呼吸器につながれた。
   _____

4. Lew's aunt's immune system responded well to the SARS infection.
   ルーの叔母さんの免疫システムは SARS 感染に対してよく抵抗した。
   _____

raise a red flag: 警鐘を鳴らす

Part 3: Listening to Medical News

Chapter 8 Listening to Medical News (3)

POINT ☞ 一般向けニュース番組で取り上げられた医療トピックを聴き，そこで使われている表現を学ぼう。

Listening

Heart Test

Before Listening 下記の医学用語は英語で何というでしょうか？ 本文中から探してみましょう。

1. 心臓病　　　　　　＿＿＿＿＿＿＿＿
2. 心臓発作　　　　　＿＿＿＿＿＿＿＿
3. 症状　　　　　　　＿＿＿＿＿＿＿＿
4. 炎症　　　　　　　＿＿＿＿＿＿＿＿
5. 冠状動脈　　　　　＿＿＿＿＿＿＿＿
6. 心臓病専門医　　　＿＿＿＿＿＿＿＿

First Listening 下線部を聴き取り，記入してみましょう。

Elizabeth Vargas: We have news about heart disease tonight. It is (1) ＿＿＿＿ ＿＿＿＿ ＿＿＿＿ ＿＿＿＿ ＿＿＿＿ in this country. Tragically many people suffer fatal heart attacks even after receiving a clean bill of health. A simple, but not widely known test can help prevent some of these sudden deaths. It can cost as little as 10 dollars. Here's our medical

fatal: 致死性の，致命的な

sudden death: 突然死

editor, Dr. Tim Johnson.

Dr. Tim Johnson: Half of all heart attacks this year will happen to people with normal cholesterol levels. (2) _____ _____ _____ _____ _____ _____ _____ _____ .

Dr. Richard Fleming, Author of "Stop Inflammation Now": Half the people who have heart disease find out that they have a heart problem by dropping dead. That's the first symptom they have.

Dr. Tim Johnson: But now there is a simple blood test that may save lives. It can detect hidden inflammation that may lead to heart attacks and the test can raise the red flag early in heart disease while there is still time (3) _____ _____ _____ _____ . The blood test is known as the CRP test. It's simple and it's cheap. CRP stands for C-reactive protein, which is the protein made in our body in response to any kind of inflammation. The super-sensitive CRP test can detect inflammation in the coronary arteries. So how did CRP become a major player in the fight against America's number 1 killer, heart disease? The answer can be found here, in the lab of Dr. Paul Ridker, a cardiologist at Boston's Brigham and Women's Hospital. He remembers his first big study on CRP in 1996 when he realized his research team had hit a home run.

Dr. Paul Ridker, Brigham and Women's Hospital: And it was an extraordinary revelation because we understood in a matter of minutes we had a better way of (4) _____ _____ _____ _____ .

Dr. Tim Johnson: Dr. Ridker believes that inflammation is

inflammation: 炎症

raise the red flag: 警鐘を鳴らす（p. 73 の red flags went off も参照）

C-reactive protein (CRP): C 反応性蛋白

coronary artery: 冠状動脈

lab (= laboratory)

the actual trigger that sets off most heart attacks. That's why having a high CRP (5) _____ _____ _____ _____ _____ _____ _____ _____ .

Dr. Paul Ridker: We've been telling patients with low cholesterol for years they're not at risk. That's just not the case.

Dr. Tim Johnson: Fortunately, (6) _____ _____ _____ _____ _____ _____ which of these people might be at risk.

Dr. Timothy Johnson, ABC News.

Heart Test (ABC News, April 16, 2004)
Reprinted with permission.

Second Listening　本文の内容と一致するものには **T**，一致しないものには **F** を付けてみましょう。

1. Half the people who have heart disease do not realize that they have a heart problem.
   心臓病を持つ人の半数は，自分が心臓に問題を抱えていることに気がつかない。　_____

2. The CRP test can detect hidden inflammation that can lead to heart attacks.
   CRP 検査は心臓発作につながる恐れのある，隠れた炎症を探り出すことができる。　_____

3. Dr. Paul Ridker and his research team hit a home run at a stadium in Boston.
   Dr. Paul Ridker と彼の研究チームはボストンのスタジア

ムでホームランを打った。　　　　　　_____

4. Patients with low cholesterol do not have to worry about heart attacks when their CRP score is high.
コレステロール値の低い患者さんは，CRPの検査値が高いと心臓発作の心配をする必要がない。　_____

Listening

Growing Arteries

Before Listening 下記の医学用語は英語で何というでしょうか？ 本文中から探してみましょう。

1. 最先端の医療　　　　　　　　_____
2. 〔締めつけられるような〕胸痛　_____
3. 血流　　　　　　　　　　　　_____
4. 手術　　　　　　　　　　　　_____
5. 遺伝子組換え蛋白〔質〕　　　_____
6. 糖尿病　　　　　　　　　　　_____

First Listening 下線部を聴き取り，記入してみましょう。

Peter Jennings: Finally from us this evening, "Medicine on the Cutting Edge." More than 6 million Americans suffer from angina or (1)_____ _____ _____ _____ _____ _____ _____ _____ _____ to the heart. We've done reports on a variety of treatments, which work for some people but not for others. Bypasses, stents, and things like that.

stent: ステント（心筋梗塞の治療などで，再発防止のために血管の中に入れる金属製の筒）

Tonight we report about doctors at the University of Cincinnati, who are providing (2) _____ _____ _____ _____ in a very new way.

Here's ABC's Barry Serafin.

Barry Serafin: Despite three heart operations including a quadruple bypass, Cincinnati mail carrier, James Duke said he felt like an elephant was on his chest.

James Duke: Constantly hurt, I'd be at home ... I know, I wanna get out and walk in a park and stuff like. I couldn't do it because I get really tired.

Barry Serafin: But since receiving (3) _____ _____ _____ _____ _____ _____ _____ , his pain is gone.

James Duke: Now I really feel great.

Barry Serafin: Duke was one of the first heart patients in the country to be treated with (4) _____ _____ _____ _____ _____ _____ _____ - _____ _____ . The genetically engineered protein is (5) _____ _____ _____ _____ _____ . Within days a network of new vessels begins to grow around the blockage, increasing the blood supply. Dr. Lynne Wagoner showed us the changes in one patient's heart.

Dr. Lynne Wagoner, The University Hospital, Cincinnati: We see a small, narrow main artery and not very many secondary and tertiary arteries. This is after the treatment. What we're now seeing is new blood vessels growing here off the end of this artery...

Barry Serafin: And the patients themselves...

Dr. Lynne Wagoner: Symptomatically they are improved within a couple of weeks of the treatment.

quadruple: 四重の

tertiary: 第3の

Chapter 8　Medical News (3)

Barry Serafin: Just ask Constance Donley.

Constance Donley: Oh, I feel wonderful. I've never felt so good in the last five years.

Barry Serafin: The (6) _____ _____ _____ _____ _____ _____ _____ _____ , but doctors already see potential in other cases where the blood supply needs a boost, such as strokes and diabetes.

stroke: 卒中

Dr. Lynne Wagoner: It's a very exciting, promising treatment for patients both of heart disease and with other cardiovascular diseases.

cardiovascular: 心臓血管の

Barry Serafin: Tests have only been underway in this country for six months on a handful of patients. If they pan out, the treatment could be available in three to four years.

Barry Serafin, ABC News, Washington.

Growing Arteries (ABC News, May 12, 2004)
Reprinted with permission.

Second Listening　本文の内容と一致するものには **T**，一致しないものには **F** を付けてみましょう。

1. More than 6 million Americans suffer from severe chest pains.
   600万人以上のアメリカ人が激しい胸痛に苦しんでいる。　_____

2. Mr. Duke's chest pain was caused by an elephant.
   デュークさんの胸痛は象が原因だった。　_____

3. Mr. Duke was treated with a protein that can grow arteries.

   デュークさんは動脈を新生する蛋白質による治療を受けた。　　　　　　　　　　　　　　　　　＿＿＿

4. This new treatment could be available in three to four years if the experiments are successful.

   この新しい治療法は，実験が成功すれば，3～4年で利用できるだろう。　　　　　　　　　　　　　＿＿＿

Part 4
Learning Medical Expressions

Part 4: Learning Medical Expressions

Chapter 9 Expressions to Describe Signs and Symptoms

> **POINT** ☞
> 1. 医師が患者さんに問診するときにしばしば登場する「訴え」(complaints)や「症状」(symptoms)の口語的英語表現を身に付けましょう。
> 2. 患者あるいは医師になったつもりで，クリニックでの実際の英会話を体験してみましょう。

Reading

At an outpatient clinic: A case of digestive problems

Doctor: Hello, Mr. John Bush. I'm Dr. Yokota. It's nice weather today, isn't it?

Mr. Bush: It is, Doctor. Not too chilly, not too warm.

Doctor: Well, what seems to be the trouble today?

Mr. Bush: I have heartburn. I also get nausea on and off without vomiting.

Doctor: Well, when did you first notice the problem?

Mr. Bush: It must have been about 6 months ago when I first noticed it. It seems to have gotten worse these last two weeks. That's why I came to see you.

Doctor: Do you have a stomachache?

Mr. Bush: No, I don't have any other special pain. It's just an obstinate heartburn.

Doctor: So you don't have a stomachache, do you? Okay. I'd like you to describe your symptoms in more detail. Does this heartburn condition run in your family?

Mr. Bush: Not that I know of.

Doctor: Do any particular foods bring on your heartburn?

Mr. Bush: Well, maybe some spicy foods seem to have a

COLUMN

初診の患者さんに相対するときの心得(1)

まず，医師は初対面の患者に笑顔で挨拶をして自己紹介をし，目の前にいる患者さんを full name で呼んで本人に間違いないことを確認すること(identification)から診察を始めます。何事も first impression が大切であり，初診の際は特に時間をかけて患者さんの主訴(chief complaint)をしっかり聞くことが大切である。また，患者さんやその家族との会話ではいわゆる専門用語(medical jargon)よりも普通の話し言葉で相手に理解できるように話し，good communication を図ることが大切です。医学の専門家である前に臨床医は good communicator でなければなりません。

(→ 97 頁の COLUMN へ続く)

日本語訳

初診外来にて：消化器病の症例

医師：こんにちは，ジョン・ブッシュさんですね。横田と申します。今日は良い天気ですね。

患者：そうですね，先生。寒くもなく，暑くもなく。

医師：さて，今日はどうなさったのですか？

患者：胸やけがします。実際に吐きはしませんが，ときどき吐き気がします。

医師：そうですか。最初にその症状に気づいたのはいつですか？

患者：最初に気がついたのは確か6ヵ月ほど前です。それがここ2週間調子が悪くなってきたような気がして，それで先生に診ていただきにきたのです。

医師：腹痛はありませんか？

患者：いいえ，特に他の痛みはありません。ちょっとしつこい胸やけだけなのです。

医師：腹痛はないのですね。これはよしと。症状についてもっと詳しく話してほしいのですが… このような胸やけの症状がご家族内で遺伝的に受け継がれているということはありますか？

患者：知るかぎりではないと思います。

医師：食べると特に胸やけのするものはありますか？

患者：そうですねぇ，たぶん香辛料の効いた食べ物で悪くなるよ

bad effect.

Doctor: How about your bowel movements? Have you noticed any color change in your stool?

Mr. Bush: Actually, I suffer from constipation and diarrhea alternately. And my stool is occasionally black lately. I don't feel any pain, though.

After the physical examination:

Doctor: Well, I think we need to do some tests, Mr. Bush. First, I'd like you to provide us with a sample of your stool. Let's confirm whether or not it contains any blood. You can take this container. Put the sample in it and bring it to us tomorrow morning.

Mr. Bush: Okay, Doctor, but what does it mean if there is blood in my stool? Is it serious? Should I worry?

Doctor: Well, Mr. Bush, there are several possibilities of gastrointestinal disease but I would rather discuss it after getting the results of the test. Okay, Mr. Bush? I will prescribe some antacids today. Take them for a week as the label says. Do you have any more questions?

Well then, I'll see you in a week. I'd like you to make the next appointment at the reception desk.

Mr. Bush: I understand, Doctor. I'll do what you want. Thank you, Dr. Yokota. I'll see you next week.

Doctor: Take care of yourself, Mr. Bush.

うです。

医師：便通はどうですか？ 便の色に変化はありませんでしたか？

患者：実は，便秘と下痢が交互にくるのに悩んでいます。また，最近たまには便が黒いことがあります。別に何の痛みも感じませんけど。

一通り診察をすませた後で：

医師：さて，ブッシュさん，いくつか追加検査が必要だと思います。まず便検査用の検体を持ってきて欲しいのです。便に血液が混じっているかどうかを確かめましょう。この容器を持ち帰り，少量の便を入れて明日午前中に持参してください。

患者：わかりました。でも，もし便に血が混じっていたら，それはどういうことなのでしょうか？ 大変なことで，心配しなければいけないのでしょうか？

医師：ブッシュさん，いくつかの胃腸の病気の可能性がありますが，それは便検査の結果が出てからお話しようと思いますが…。よろしいでしょうか，ブッシュさん。今日は制酸薬を出しておきましょう。これを1週間，ラベルの指示に従って服用してください。他に何かご質問はあるでしょうか？ では，1週間後に再診にしましょう。受付で予約を取ってください。いいですね，ブッシュさん。

患者：はい，わかりました。おっしゃるようにします。先生，どうもありがとうございました。では来週参ります。

医師：お大事に，ブッシュさん。

Word Check

■症状

- **heartburn** [hάɚtbɚ̀ːn, hάːtbɚ̀ːn] *n.* 胸やけ

  （上腹部や胸骨下の灼熱感のような痛み。胃酸が食道内に逆流して生じる食道炎に伴う症状であることが多い。heart + burn ではあるが，心臓が原因で起こる症状ではない。専門用語で pyrosis [pàɪ(ə)róʊsɪs] ともいう。【語源分析】pyrosis → pyro-(熱，火) + -sis(…の状態)→焼けるように熱く感じる状態→胸やけ）

- **nausea** [nɔ́ːziə, -ʒə, -siə, -ʃə] *n.* 吐き気，嘔気，悪心

  （ギリシャ語 naus[船]が語源で，本来は「船酔い（seasickness）」の意味。形容詞は nauseous [nɔ́ːʃəs, -ʒiəs, -siəs] で，feel nauseous[吐き気がする] = feel nauseated）

- **vomiting** [vάmɪtɪŋ, vɔ́m-] *n.* 嘔吐

  （悪心[nausea]を伴う場合，しばしば nausea and vomiting[カルテには略して N & V と表現することがある）

- **stomachache** [stʌ́məkèɪk] *n.* 腹痛，胃痛

  （stomach(胃) + ache(痛み)→胃痛であるが，胃だけでなく，腹部の痛みを表すのにも使われる。専門用語では gastralgia [gæstrǽldʒə] とか gastrodynia [gæstroʊdάɪniə] と記載する。【語源分析】gastralgia → gastr-(胃) + -algia(疼痛)→胃痛；gastrodynia → gastro-(胃) + -dynia(疼痛)→胃痛）

■基本的な医学用語

- **symptom** [sím(p)təm] *n.* 症状，徴候

  （【語源分析】symptom → sym- (= syn- 共に，一緒に) + ptom (落ちるもの)→一緒になって落ちてくるもの→病気の症状などが一緒に出現すること→症状）

- **bowel movement** 便通，排便

  （直訳すれば「腸の運動」であり，その結果として排便が起

豆知識

stomachache の文字通りの訳は「胃痛」ですが，もっとおおざっぱに「腹痛」を表すこともあります。医学的に stomach は「胃」ですが，一般的には「腹部」を意味することがあるのです。また口語では bellyache や tummyache も「腹痛」として用いられることがあります。

こるのだから合理的な表現。日本語の「お通じ」に近いニュアンスである。「お通じ［便通］は正常ですか。」は "Do you have a normal bowel movement." といえばよい。複数形 bowel movements で用いられることもしばしばある。また，時に英語では「糞便」そのものを bowel movement ということがある。B.M. と略される。専門用語としては defecation [dèfikéɪʃən] がある。【語源分析】defecation → de-（離れて，脱）+ fec（= feces 糞便）+ -ation（…すること）→便を直腸から体外に出し除去すること→排便）

- **stool** [stúːl] *n.* 大便

  （最も一般的な「便」を表現する単語。他に feces [físiːz] や，小児科領域で「うんち」に相当する小児語 poo-poo [púːpúː] などがある）

- **constipation** [kɑ̀nstəpéɪʃən, kɔ̀n-] *n.* 便秘

  （【語源分析】constipation → con-（一緒に，まとまって）+ stipation（詰め込むこと）→便が腸内に一緒にまとまって詰め込まれた状態になること→便が腸の中に留まった状態→便秘）

- **diarrhea** [dàɪəríːə] *n.* 下痢

  （英国式のスペリングでは diarrhoea となる。【語源分析】diarrhea → dia-（…を通して，貫通して）+ -rrhea（流れること）→直腸や肛門を通して便が流れ出ること→下痢）

- **physical examination**　身体検査（＝診察）

  （「理学的検査」ともいわれるが，正しくは「身体検査」。狭い意味での「診察」に相当する。しばしば会話では physical exam と略していわれる）

- **gastrointestinal** [gæ̀strouintéstənl] *a.* 胃腸の

  （gastroenteric [gæ̀strouentérɪk] と同じ意味。gastrointestinal tract で「消化管」。【語源分析】gastrointestinal → gastro-（胃）+ intestinal（腸の）→胃腸の；gastroenteric → gastro-（胃）+ enteric（腸の）→胃腸の）

■ **動詞表現**

- **get worse**　悪化する
- **run in one's family (run in the family)**　家系的に生じている，血筋として起こっている

  (遺伝性疾患があるかどうかを尋ねるときのフレーズ)

- **have a bad effect**　悪影響がある

  (逆の表現は have a good effect で「有効である，よい影響がある」)

- **suffer from ...**　…で悩む，…で苦しむ，…を患う

  (病状を訴える際に「つらい思いをしている」というニュアンスを出すためにしばしば用いられる)

■ **その他**

- **on and off**　断続的に，出たり出なかったり
- **two weeks** *n.*　2週間

  (イギリス英語では fortnight [fɔ́ːtnàɪt, fɔ́ːt-] ともいうが，アメリカ英語では fortnight よりも two weeks の方が一般的。【語源分析】fortnight → fourteen + night = 14 夜 = 2 週間)

- **in more detail**　もっと詳しく
- **How about ...?**　「…についてはどうですか？」と特定の事項に関して相手の考えを尋ねる際に用いる表現で，応用範囲が広い。What about ...? でも同様の表現ができる。

Word Study

■ **symptoms** と **signs** の相違は？

　患者さん自身が訴える自覚症状のことを symptom といい，医学的には symptoms を「症候」と訳すこともあります。また特に患者さんが医療を求めてやって来た理由になる主な症状を「主訴 (chief complaint)」といいます。一方，sign は医師が診察の結果として見出す客観的なもので，「徴候」と訳しま

す。すなわち symptoms and signs で「症候と徴候」となります。しかし，一般的な口語的表現としては「症状と所見」という意味になります。また，英語としては signs and symptoms という語順の方がより多く使われています。患者さんの訴えから symptoms を的確に捉え，診察を通して正しい signs を得ることが，初診時の最も重要な医療行為です。

単数形か複数形かについては，しばしば複数の症状が存在するので，通常は symptoms and signs と複数形で覚えておけばよいでしょう。また clinical findings（臨床所見）という類似表現も用いられます。

■「症状」に関する表現

患者さんの訴え，すなわち chief complaint を把握するために，"Well, what seems to be the problem today?" という表現が用いられていますが，"What's the problem?" という直接的表現でも用は足りますし，実際の会話ではもう少しなめらかでくだけた表現が好まれます。具体的には "What's the problem today?" のように today を付けたり，"What seems to be the problem?" あるいは "Well, what seems to be the problem today?" のようにことばを足すことで，気持ちのこもった対面会話らしい表現になります。

> 「今日はどうされたのですか？」の例
> ・What seems to be the problem today?
> ・What seems to be the trouble today?
> ・What can I do for you today?
> ・What's the problem today?
> ・What's the trouble today?
> ・What's the matter with you today?
> ・What's wrong with you today?
> ・What brought you here today?
> ・How can I help you today?

その他にも直接的な表現として，"What kind of symptoms do you have?"（どんな症状があるのですか？）などを使ってもよいでしょう。

■ 「症状」を表す用語

症状のうち非常に多いのが頭痛や腹痛，腰痛，胸部痛，そして外傷を負ったときの「痛み」です。何らかの「痛み」があるから医療機関を受診するのだともいえます。「痛み」についての表現は特に重要であり，後の章で詳しく学ぶことにしましょう。

痛み以外の主な症状を表す単語には以下のようなものがあります。

- ☐ fever [fí:vɚ, -və] 発熱
- ☐ chills [tʃilz] 寒気（形容詞は chilly [tʃíli]）
- ☐ cough [kɔ́:f] 咳
- ☐ nausea [nɔ́:ziə, -ʒə, -siə, -ʃə] 吐き気，嘔気，悪心
- ☐ vomiting [vámitiŋ, vɔ́m-] 嘔吐
- ☐ diarrhea [dàɪərí:ə] 下痢
- ☐ constipation [kànstəpéɪʃən] 便秘
- ☐ bleeding [blí:dɪŋ]
    hemorrhage [hém(ə)rɪdʒ] 出血
- ☐ swelling [swéliŋ] 腫れ
- ☐ edema [idí:mə] 浮腫
- ☐ itching [ítʃiŋ] かゆみ，掻痒
- ☐ numbness [nʌ́mnis] しびれ
- ☐ heartburn [háɚtbɚ:n, há:tbə:n] 胸やけ
- ☐ runny nose [rʌ́ni nóuz] 鼻水（My nose is running としても「鼻水」の意）
- ☐ runny ear [rʌ́ni iɚ] 耳だれ
- ☐ boil [bɔ́ɪl] できもの

- ☐ allergy [ǽlədʒi] アレルギー
- ☐ hearing loss; impaired hearing; be hard of hearing 難聴
- ☐ phlegm [flém]; sputum [sp(j)ú:təm] 痰（sputum の方が専門用語的なニュアンスがある）
- ☐ dizziness [dízinis] めまい全般を表すあいまいな表現
- ☐ giddiness [gídinis] めまい（dizziness よりさらにあいまい）
- ☐ vertigo [və́:rtəgòu] めまい（はっきりとした回転性のめまい）
- ☐ hangover 二日酔い
- ☐ insomnia [ɪnsámniə, -sóm-]; difficulty sleeping; sleeping disturbance 不眠
- ☐ weight loss; loss of weight 体重減少
- ☐ poor appetite [— ǽpətàɪt]; loss of appetite 食欲不振
- ☐ rash [rǽʃ] 皮疹
- ☐ hot flash [— flʌ́ʃ]; flushed face 顔面紅潮
- ☐ anemia [əní:miə] 貧血

■会話表現

1. I have ...

ある症状にかかっていると英語で表現したいときには，単純に "I have ..." の "..." のところに症状や病気を表す名詞を入れます。これを"**病気の have**"あるいは"**症状の have**"などと称して覚えてもよいでしょう。例えば「熱がある」なら "I have a fever." といえばよいし，また「頭痛がする」や「お腹が痛む」なら，それぞれ "I have a headache.", "I have a stomachache." といえばよいのです。また I have got ...（= I've got ...）という表現も頻用されます。例えば，I have a cold. = I have got a cold. = I've got a cold. のような関係が成り立ちます。

2. Have you ever had ...?（これまでに起こったことを尋ねる場合）

"..."のところに症状や病名を入れると，病歴聴取の際に有効な応用ができます。

- ☐ Have you ever had ...?
  （…を持ったことがありますか？＝…を経験したことがありますか？）
- ☐ Have you ever experienced ...?
  （…を経験したことがありますか？）
- ☐ Have you ever suffered from ...?
  （…にかかったことがありますか？）
- ☐ Have you noticed ...?
  （…に気付いたことはありますか？）

3. Do you have ...?（習慣的な症状や状態や現在起こっている症状を尋ねる場合）
- ☐ Do you have any difficulty in ...?
  （…で困難を感じますか？）
- ☐ Do you have any trouble with ...?
  （…に問題はありますか？）

4. 視力や聴覚が正常かどうかを尋ねる場合の代表的例文
- ☐ Can you see and hear all right?
  （ちゃんと見たり聞いたりすることができますか？）
- ☐ Do you see and hear all right?
  （ちゃんとものが見えたり聞こえたりしていますか？）
- ☐ Do you have any trouble with your vision or hearing?
  （視力や聴力に問題がありますか？）

「視力」は英語で visual acuity といいますが，よく見えないと

きには簡単に "I can't see too well" あるいは "I have a poor vision" などといえば通じます。ぼんやりと見えるのなら "I have a blurred vision" や "I have a hazy vision" などといいます。完全に見えなくなれば loss of vision や blind の状態なので，"I have a loss of vision" や "I am blind" といいます。また，物がだぶって見えるかどうか尋ねる場合には，"Do you see double?" や "Do you have any double vision?" あるいは単に "Any double vision?" と訊けばよいでしょう。ちなみに専門用語としての「複視」は diplopia [dɪpóupiə] といいます。

■ 冠詞の用法

　冠詞が要るのか要らないのか，要るとすれば "a" か "an" か，それとも "the" か？ 医療英会話の現場ではその使い方に苦労してきた医師も少なくないので，これに関しても少し説明を加えておきましょう。

　例えば，「私は風邪をひいている」は "I have a cold" で，風邪は必ず "a cold" となり，"I have cold" としてはいけません。しかし，「頭痛がする」という場合，"I have a headache" と頭痛を "a headache" とするのが普通であるけれども，では "I have headache" としては絶対にいけないのかどうか？ 逆に，「下痢がある，下痢である」あるいは「便秘がある，便秘である」なら普通それぞれ "I have diarrhea," "I have constipation" といいますが，これを "I have a diarrhea" あるいは "I have a constipation" としてはいけないのか？ *Reading* にも出てきましたが「胸やけがする」は "I have heartburn" が普通よく耳にしたり見たりする表現ですが，"I have a heartburn" としてはいけないのか？ このような冠詞に関する疑問に対して，どこでも常に通用するような歯切れのよい回答を出すのは難しいのです。

　結論からいえば，仮に文法的に間違っていなくてもネイテ

ィブの英米人が日常どれをよく使っているかで標準的な表現形式が決まってくるともいえます。けれども以下のようなおおまかなルールを覚えておくと，役に立つでしょう。

冠詞の使い方についての3つの原則

① 軽い症状で，日常的に話題になるようなものには"**a**"を付けます。

I have a cold.

I have a headache.

My child has a rash over his body.

② 感染性の強い病気などには"**the**"を付けます。

I have the flu.

I have the chickenpox.

I have the sniffles.

She had the hives.

③ 重い病気，子供の病気，アレルギー症状には冠詞を付けません。

My father has cancer.

My grandmother has Alzheimer's disease.

Many people have hay fever in springtime.

He sometimes has diarrhea.

Chapter 9 Expressions of Signs and Symptoms

■ **bring on ...**（症状の増悪因子について確認する表現）

"Do any particular foods bring on your heartburn?" のように，"bring on ..." で「…を起こす，…を惹起する」と表現するのが簡明です。同様の意味を "Are there any particular foods that make your heartburn worse?" と表現することもできます。一般的に「症状が悪化する」は make one's symptom(s) worse といいます。逆に「症状が良くなる」は make one's symptom(s) better と表現することを覚えておけば，応用が利きます。「何か症状を改善するものがありますか？」と訊く場合には，"Are there any particular things that make your symptoms better?" といいます。

COLUMN

初診の患者さんに相対するときの心得(2)

「臨床的に患者さんを診る」ということは，①まず問診によって主訴を明らかにし，②その背景となる既往歴(medical history)や家族歴(family history)，生活習慣(lifestyle, living habits)や他の合併症(coexisting illness)の有無，あるいはすでに受けている治療などについて整理して，③身体検査を実施し，④さらに必要な臨床検査を選択して，⑤その結果を踏まえて診断を下し，それに対して適切な治療を実施するということです。一連の問診のことを英語で history taking といい，その良し悪しがその後の患者さんの命運を決するほどの意味をもつ最も重要な臨床医の技能です。

　このプロセスはヒポクラテスの時代から "art" と称されてきました。ヒポクラテスの言葉として残されている "*ars longa vita brevis*"（ラテン語）の英訳が "Art is long, life is short." です。この場合の art の元の意味は「医術」「医師としての精進の道」です。医療の科学的な側面の他に，心理面や社会的側面において患者さんとのラポール（"rapport" フランス語：協調的あるいは共感的な関係）を築いていくことが重要です。

　問診時の質問形式としては，一般的には "What seems to be the trouble?" のように相手に語らせる open questions から多くの情報が得られます。また情報を整理するためには必要に応じて Yes や No で答えてもらう closed questions も必要となります。この2つの質問形式を使い分けることが必要です。84ページの Reading 中にある "So you don't have a stomachache, do you?" のような付加疑問文は，あいまいさを減らすことができるので便利ですが，使いすぎると相手に不快感を与えることもあります。

　実際の英語圏での診察現場においては，医師は患者さんの名前を何度も会話に盛り込み，さらに Well, Now, Good, Okay, All right などの語句を頻繁に使用しています。適切に用いると，うまく話の流れをつくったり，患者さんに安心感を与えたりするのに役立ちます。これらの言葉を会話から取り去ると，冷ややかな感じの医師−患者関係(doctor−patient relationship)になりそうです。

Exercise

1. 医師が患者さんに病状を尋ねるときの「今日はどうされましたか？」にあたる表現を英語で少なくとも3通り書き出し，音読しましょう。

   _____

   _____

   _____

2. 患者さんが症状を訴える表現を学ぶことにしましょう。次の例にならって①から⑧の場合の症状を表現する英語を書きましょう。

   例1：最近になって難聴となってきた場合
   → I'm a little hard of hearing these days.
   （このごろ少し耳が遠くなりました。）

   例2：視力が徐々に低下している場合の患者さんの主訴
   → My eyesight is gradually worsening.
   （視力が徐々に悪くなっているような気がします。）

   ① ここ2～3日，下痢(diarrhea)に悩んでいる場合。

   → _____

   ② めまい(名詞 dizziness，形容詞は dizzy)がする場合。

   → _____

   ③ 皮疹(skin rash あるいは単に rash)が出てきた場合。

   → _____

   ④ 発熱(fever)がある場合。

   → _____

⑤ お腹がむかむか(nauseous あるいは nauseated)して食欲不振(poor appetite, loss of appetite)になった場合。

→ _____

⑥ ものが二重に見える(see double)場合。

→ _____

⑦ ここ2週間(two weeks あるいは fortnight)くらい胸やけ(heartburn)を自覚している場合。

→ _____

⑧ 「あなたの症状を悪化させたり，改善させたりする何か特別な要因がありますか？」と尋ねる場合。

→ _____

3. 次の各症状に相当する英単語を書きましょう。

吐き気，嘔気　　　_____

胸やけ　　　　　　_____

鼻水　　　　　　　_____

便秘　　　　　　　_____

下痢　　　　　　　_____

咳　　　　　　　　_____

はれもの，できもの　_____

むくみ(浮腫)　　　_____

発熱　　　　　　　_____

アレルギー　　　　_____

難聴　　　　　＿＿＿＿＿＿＿＿＿＿＿＿＿＿＿＿＿＿＿

寒気　　　　　＿＿＿＿＿＿＿＿＿＿＿＿＿＿＿＿＿＿＿

痰　　　　　　＿＿＿＿＿＿＿＿＿＿＿＿＿＿＿＿＿＿＿

めまい　　　　＿＿＿＿＿＿＿＿＿＿＿＿＿＿＿＿＿＿＿

二日酔い　　　＿＿＿＿＿＿＿＿＿＿＿＿＿＿＿＿＿＿＿

食欲低下　　　＿＿＿＿＿＿＿＿＿＿＿＿＿＿＿＿＿＿＿

かゆみ，掻痒感　＿＿＿＿＿＿＿＿＿＿＿＿＿＿＿＿＿＿＿

不眠　　　　　＿＿＿＿＿＿＿＿＿＿＿＿＿＿＿＿＿＿＿

体重減少　　　＿＿＿＿＿＿＿＿＿＿＿＿＿＿＿＿＿＿＿

出血　　　　　＿＿＿＿＿＿＿＿＿＿＿＿＿＿＿＿＿＿＿

4. 「いつからその症状が始まりましたか？」と質問するときの英語表現を少なくとも3通り書き出し音読しましょう。

　　＿＿＿＿＿＿＿＿＿＿＿＿＿＿＿＿＿＿＿＿＿＿＿＿＿＿＿＿＿＿＿＿＿＿＿

　　＿＿＿＿＿＿＿＿＿＿＿＿＿＿＿＿＿＿＿＿＿＿＿＿＿＿＿＿＿＿＿＿＿＿＿

　　＿＿＿＿＿＿＿＿＿＿＿＿＿＿＿＿＿＿＿＿＿＿＿＿＿＿＿＿＿＿＿＿＿＿＿

5. 診察終了後の別れ際の挨拶の表現には日本語でも「お大事に」などがあります。英語では何といいますか。

　　＿＿＿＿＿＿＿＿＿＿＿＿＿＿＿＿＿＿＿＿＿＿＿＿＿＿＿＿＿＿＿＿＿＿＿

　　＿＿＿＿＿＿＿＿＿＿＿＿＿＿＿＿＿＿＿＿＿＿＿＿＿＿＿＿＿＿＿＿＿＿＿

Part 4: Learning Medical Expressions

Chapter 10 Expressions to Describe Vital Signs

> **POINT** ☞ 医療場面で患者さんからの情報を得る際の最も基本となる "vital signs" に関する英語表現や語彙を学習しましょう。

Reading

In the ER: Mr. Smith was brought to the ER by ambulance. He is suffering from an ongoing chest pain.

Mr. Smith: (The patient seems to be upset about his chest pain.) I must be having a heart attack! The pain is killing me. What am I going to do?

(A doctor comes to see him.)

Doctor: Can you hear me now, Mr. Smith?

Mr. Smith: Oh, yes. I am having a pain in my chest. It's (a) severe pain. And I feel nauseated. Did I have a heart attack? Am I going to die, Doc?

Doctor: Please calm down. Don't panic. Just calm down and try to relax. Now, I'm going to ask you some very important questions, ... All right? When did this pain start bothering you?

Mr. Smith: About half an hour ago. It came suddenly, without warning.

Doctor: Have you had these same symptoms before?

Mr. Smith: Well, yes. I've had chest pain once a month or so lately. The pain was usually less severe and didn't last so long. Doc, I'm afraid I'm getting even

COLUMN

Vital Signs

"vital signs"は「生命徴候」と和訳されることもあるが，医療現場では，「ヴァイタル（バイタル）サイン」としてすでに日常的な職業用語として定着しています。4つの客観的徴候，すなわち体温（body temperature），脈拍数（pulse rate），血圧（blood pressure），そして呼吸数（respiratory rate）のセットとして用いられることが一般的で，ほとんど常に "vital signs" と複数形で用いられます（この4つに意識レベル consciousness を含めて5つとする場合もあります）。

これらのどれかに異常があれば，それは生命維持にとって重大な問題があることを示しています。重症患者の場合，特に "vital signs" の変化を経時的に観察することが重要です。

日本語訳

救急外来（emergency room; ER）に胸痛を訴えて苦しむ高齢男性患者が救急車で来院した場面

患者：（周囲にかまわず，かなり取り乱して…）心臓発作に違いない。苦しくて死にそうだ。どうすればいいんだろう？

（医師がやって来て）

医師：さあ，私のいうことがわかりますか？

患者：ええ，わかります。ひどく胸が痛いんです。それに吐き気もあります。心臓発作でしょうか？ 先生，私は死んでしまうんでしょうか？

医師：慌てないで。さあ落ち着いてください。今からとても大切な質問をします，いいですね。いつから苦しくなったのですか？

患者：30分くらい前です。急に起こりました。

医師：以前にも同じ症状がありましたか。

患者：ええ，ありました。最近では月に1回くらい胸痛がしてました。これまではもっと痛くなくて短かったのです。先生，ちょっと気分が悪くなってます。吐きそうだ。先生，何とかして

worse now. I'm going to throw up ... Please do something for me, Doc!

Doctor: All right, all right. Let me quickly examine you, now. I'd like to check your pulse and blood pressure. Your pulse rate is 80, regular. And your blood pressure is 162/90, a bit higher than the normal range. (The doctor is saying to himself ... The respiratory rate is 22 and the oxygen saturation is 90%.)

Mr. Smith: Anything wrong?

Doctor: We are just checking the basic vital signs. Now, let me take your temperature. Put this thermometer under your arm. (after a minute or so) Your temperature is 36.5 °C. That's within normal limits.

After further physical examinations:

Doctor: Well, you have a strong possibility of having a heart attack, or medically known as an acute myocardial infarction. We need to carry out further tests such as ECG, cardiac ultrasound, and blood testing to confirm the diagnosis.

Mr. Smith: Is it serious, Doc?

Doctor: Well, don't worry too much. We are doing everything possible. Whatever the diagnosis, your present condition requires hospitalization (your present condition requires that you be hospitalized) . Okay, Mr. Smith?

ください。

医師：わかりました。では，急いで診察しましょう。脈拍と血圧のチェックをします。脈拍数は80で不整なし。血圧は162の90でちょっと高めですね。
（患者の胸の動きを見ながら独り言のように）呼吸数は22回で，酸素飽和度が90％。

患者：何かおかしいところがわかりましたか？
医師：基本的なヴァイタルサインをチェックしているのです。体温を測りましょう。この体温計を脇の下に入れてください。（しばらくして）体温は36.5℃で，正常範囲です。

その他の診察を終えて
医師：どうも心臓発作というか，医学的にいえば急性心筋梗塞を起こしている可能性が高いと思われます。診断を確定するために心電図，心エコー，血液検査などの追加検査が必要です。

患者：重症ですか？
医師：あまり心配しすぎないでください。できることはすべてやっていますから。いずれにしても今の状況では入院して治療が必要です。よろしいですか，スミスさん。

Word Check

■ **vital signs** に関する用語

- **heart attack**　心臓発作

  (心筋梗塞[myocardial infarction, MI と略す]の日常的な言い方)

- **a pain in my chest**　胸痛

  (a chest pain ともいう。"a pain in one's ..." を覚えておくだけで，"..." に身体の部位名を入れれば全身のほとんどの痛みを表現することができる。「私は…が痛い」は "I have a pain in my ...." と定型的に覚えてよい)

- **feel nauseated**　吐き気がする

  (= feel nauseous; have nausea)

- **panic** [pǽnɪk] *n.* パニック，恐慌；*v.* パニックに陥る，うろたえる

  (語源はギリシャ神話にでてくる牧神 Pan に由来。Pan は突然現れて人や動物を脅かす半獣神であるとされる。日本語でも「恐慌」よりも「パニック」の方が日常会話では使用頻度が高い。"Don't panic." で「落ち着け」の意味)

- **pulse** [pʌ́ls]　脈，脈拍

  (臨床場面で pulse という場合には pulse rate (脈拍数) を意味することが多い。しばしば P と略記される)

- **blood pressure** [blʌ́d préʃɚ]　血圧

  (収縮期血圧 [systolic blood pressure] と拡張期血圧 [diastolic blood pressure] の2つの数値で表す。しばしば BP と略記される)

- **respiratory rate** [résp(ə)rətɔ̀ːri réit]　呼吸数

  (1分間の呼吸数で表す。数字だけでいうことが多いが，正確には "The respiratory rate is 22 /min." あるいは "22 breaths per minute" とすべきであろう。しかし，現実の場面では暗黙の了解と切迫した時間の流れのなかで "The

respiratory rate is ...." の "..." に数字だけが入る)
- **temperature** [témp(ə)rətʃùɚ, -tʃɚ]　温度, 体温
(状況が医療の現場であれば, body temperature とせずに temperature だけで「体温」の意味に用いる。ただ, 「熱がある」を "I have a temperature." と表現することがあるので要注意)

■ 基本的な医学用語
- **acute myocardial infarction**　急性心筋梗塞
(しばしば AMI と略される)
- **cardiac** [káɚdiæk]　*a.* 心臓の
- **diagnosis** [dàiəgnóusɪs]　診断
(【語源分析】diagnosis → dia-(…を通して, 貫通して)＋ gnosis(知っている状態)→実施した診察・検査を通して知り得た状態→診断)

■ 動詞表現
- **It's killing me.**　「そのせいで辛くてたまらない」という誇張表現
- **calm down**　落ち着く
- **try to relax**　リラックスするようにする
- **throw up**　吐く
(「吐きたくなった」という場合, しばしば "I feel like I'm going to throw up." と表現される。throw up がしばしば話し言葉の中で用いられるのに対し, vomit [vámit, vɔ́m-] は「嘔吐する」という意味で一般的ではあるが少し硬い感じがする)

■ 検査用語
- **oxygen saturation** [ɑ́ksɪdʒən sætʃuréɪʃən]　酸素飽和度
(血中の酸素飽和度をパルスオキシメータ [pulse oxime-

107

ter]という装置で，無侵襲で簡単に測定できるようになった。vital signs を得るとともに現在の救急外来では oxygen saturation もチェックすることが普通である。正常値は 95 ％以上で，90 ％以下は酸素が血中に足りないことを意味する。oxygen は化学式[chemical formula]では O_2 なので，しばしば O_2 saturation の形でも用いられる）

- **thermometer** [θərmάmətər]　温度計，体温計

  （特に clinical thermometer といわなくても，医療機関で thermometer といえば「体温計」のことである）

- **... °C** [dɪgríːz sélsiəs]　摂氏…度

  （degrees Celsius または degrees centigrade の略。米国では今でも華氏温度単位[°F: degrees Fahrenheit [dɪgríːz fǽrənhàɪt]]が用いられている。摂氏と華氏の換算式は，

  　　　　（°F − 32）× 5/9 ＝ °C

  となる[0°C = 32°F，100°C = 212°F]。ちなみに摂氏温度計は a Celsius thermometer あるいは a centigrade thermometer といい，華氏温度計は a Fahrenheit thermometer という）

- **ECG**　心電図

  （electrocardiogram [ɪlèktroukάɚdiəgræm] の略。脳波を表す electroencephalogram [ɪlèktrou-ɪnséfələgræm] の略 EEG との発音上の混同を避けるために，ECG のことを EKG と略記することもある。【語源分析】electrocardiogram → electro-（電気）+ cardio-（心臓）+ -gram（記録，図）→心臓の電気的変化の記録図→心電図）

- **ultrasound** [ʌ́ltrəsáund]　超音波，超音波検査，エコー検査

  （「超音波検査」のことは ultrasonography [ʌ̀ltrəsənɔ́grəfɪ] や echography [ekάgrəfɪ, ekɔ́-] ともいうが，ultrasound が最も日常会話的な表現である。"I had an ultrasound on my heart"[心臓の超音波検査を受けました。]【語源分析】ultrasound → ultra-（超）+ sound（音）→超音波）

■ その他
- **ER** (= emergency room)　救急救命室

  （TV ドラマの邦題である「緊急救命室」の訳も用いられている）

- **ambulance** 救急車

  （「救急車で」は by ambulance。【語源分析】ambulance → ambul(歩く，移動する) + -ance(名詞語尾)→歩き回る病院→移動式病院→救急車）

- **Doc** [dák, dɔ́k]　医師のこと。あまり上品な医師への呼びかけとは思えないが，米国でしばしば Doctor の略として会話の中で用いられている。

Word Study

■「胸痛」について

"I have a pain in my chest" が標準的な言い回し方ですが，実際の会話では "I've got a pain in my chest" という表現で使われることの方が多いようです。口語では it is は it's，I am は I'm，he is や he has は he's など，省略されることが普通です。また痛みの強さを表す場合，a severe pain(強い痛み)，a mild pain(弱い痛み)のように表現しますが，strong，weak を使うこともあります。heart attack は「心臓発作」と訳され，しばしば耳にする言葉ですが，専門用語でいえば myocardial infarction(心筋梗塞)のことです。

■「罹っている」の表現

何らかの病気に「罹（かか）っている」を表現する場合には，ほとんど have = have got を用いて表現します。

　例：I have a cold.

　　　（私はかぜを引いている。）

He's got a rash all over his body.
（彼は体中に発疹を持っている。＝彼の体中に発疹ができている。）

I have athlete's foot.
（私は水虫に罹っている。＝私は水虫だ。）

She has breast cancer.
（彼女は乳癌に罹っている。＝彼女は乳癌だ。）

He's got lung cancer.
（彼は肺癌に罹っている。）

I've got high blood pressure.
＝ I've got hypertension.
（私は高血圧だ。）

　また，以上のような「…に罹っている」という表現の多くは，suffer from ... を用いて言い換えることができます。例えば "The patient has severe obesity" = "The patient suffers from severe obesity"（その患者は重症の肥満である），"They had diabetes" = "They suffered from diabetes"（彼らは糖尿病に罹っていた）のように，have を suffer from に置き換えることが可能です。

■患者さんを落ち着かせる表現

　panic は名詞では「パニック，恐慌」ですが，動詞として使うと「うろたえる」という意味になります。"Don't panic" で「慌てないで，パニックにならないで」という表現になります。「落ち着いて」は "Calm down" や "Keep your cool" "Take it easy" と表現します。落ち着きのない患者さんに対しては，*Reading* の例文のように "Try to relax" や "Just relax" "You don't have to panic" あるいは "Just calm down" などが使えます。また "Everything is under control" などといって気を落ち着けてもらうのも一つのやり方です。

■ 症状がいつから生じたのかを尋ねる表現

"When did it start bothering you?" は，患者さんの訴える症状がいつから起きたのかを尋ねる決まり文句です。"When did it start?" あるいは "When did you first start with your symptom?" としてもかまいません。いずれも症状がいつから始まったかを直接過去形で訊く表現です。また現在完了形を用いて，"How long have you had this symptom?"（この症状はどのくらい続いていますか？）のように，どのくらいの期間ある症状が継続しているのか尋ねることによって，いつ症状が出現したかを推定することもできます。

■ vital signs をチェックするときの表現

臨床現場において，患者さんの状態を最も端的に表す客観的な基本指標が，body temperature（体温），pulse rate（脈拍数），blood pressure（血圧），respiratory rate（呼吸数）の vital signs です。vital signs をチェックする場合には，"Let me take your temperature"（体温を計らせてください），"Let me take your pulse"（脈を取らせてください），"Let me take your blood pressure"（血圧を測らせてください）のように "Let me take your ..." で表現します。ただし respiratory rate だけは客観的に胸の動きを観察して評価するので，通常は患者さんに "Let me check your respiratory rate" ということはありません。

■ 血圧値を英語で読む場合

血圧の単位は mmHg で "millimeters of mercury" と読みます。しかし，会話の中では例文 "Your blood pressure is 162/90." のように単位を省略する傾向があります。医療環境内では血圧の単位が「ミリメータ水銀柱」であることが自明なためと，単位を読むことが臨床の場に馴染まないためです。ただ同時に，お互いの単位の理解が違ったために生じた医療

事故も少なくないことも意識しておきたいものです。"162/90" の部分は "one sixty-two over ninety" と読みます。"/" は，血圧の読み方においては常に "over" と読みます。現在の定義では，血圧は 140/90 以上が高血圧とされています。

■脈拍数を英語で読む場合

pulse rate の単位は実際には beats/minute で，"/" は per [pɚː] と読みます。カルテには beats per minute の略で bpm と記載することもあります。ただし会話の中では "It's 66." とか "It's 120." のように数字だけいう場合が多いようです。

■「正常範囲内」という表現

英語で検査値などが「正常範囲内」という場合には，"within normal limits" という表現が頻用されています。カルテに記載する際にはしばしば WNL と略記され，「すべて正常範囲内」なら "all WNL" と記載されます。

■会話で用いられる英単語と医療用語との違い

一般の会話で用いられる単語と医療英語との違いを知ることも必要になります。いくつか例を示します。

一般用語			専門用語	
heart attack	心臓発作	→	myocardial infarction	心筋梗塞
high blood pressure	高血圧	→	hypertension	高血圧〔症〕
belly, stomach, tummy	腹，おなか	→	abdomen	腹，腹部
boil	おでき	→	furuncle	癤（せつ）
irregular heart beat	心拍の乱れ	→	arrhythmia	不整脈
gut, bowels	腸	→	intestines	腸，腸管
phlegm	痰	→	sputum	痰，喀痰

Exercise

1. 質問に対して英語で答えましょう。

    ① What are vital signs?

    → _____

    ② What instrument is used to measure your blood pressure?

    → _____

2. 次の日本語を英語に翻訳しましょう。

    ① 患者：私の血圧はいくつですか？

    → _____

    医師：あなたの血圧は115の65で，きわめて正常ですよ。

    → _____

    ② 患者：それで，私の脈はどうですか？問題ありませんか？

    → _____

    医師：そうですね，脈拍数は66回ですが，不整脈があります。
    　できるだけ早く心電図を取りましょう。

    → _____
    　_____

    ③ 脈を取らせてください。

    → _____

④ 血圧を測らせてください。

→ _____

⑤ 体温を測定しましょう。

→ _____

⑥ 「患者は 65 歳の男性で，息切れと咳を訴えて救急外来を受診しました。ヴァイタルサインは，体温 37.5 ℃で，脈拍数 98，血圧 160/90 で，呼吸数は毎分 24 回です。」
　（医療従事者間での伝達の際には，しばしばこのような表現が用いられる）

→ _____
　_____
　_____

COLUMN

癌はなぜカニなのか？

「癌」の英単語がcancerであることは，医療関係者以外にもよく知られています。このcancerの語源は，ギリシャ語の*karkinos*です。命名者は「医学の父」と尊敬されるヒポクラテス（Hipppocrates: 460 B.C.〜377 B.C.）です。彼は乳癌の患者の胸部を切開したとき，癌腫がカニの甲羅のように見え，その周辺にはまるでカニが脚を広げたかのように静脈が浮き上がっていたことから，乳癌を「カニのような」という意味の*karkinos*と呼んだそうです。

ギリシャ語の*karkinos*は，やがてラテン語で同義のcarcinomaに，そしてローマ帝国に支配され，それに強い影響を受けたフランス語でcancerとなり，それが英語に入ってcancerとなりました（ドイツ語では同義のder Krebs）。医学英語にはcancerと同様にギリシャ・ラテン語由来の用語がとても多いのです。

ちなみにヒポクラテスが「医学の父」と尊称されるのは，彼が何よりも臨床を重んじた医師であったからです。当時，治療困難な病気には怪しげな魔術や祈祷がよく行われていましたが，ヒポクラテスは患者のベッドサイドで，表情，脈拍，発熱などの変化を観察し，その経過を記録することによって病気の原因や治療法を考えたからです。検査法が発達した現在でも，医師は患者さんのベッドサイドに立つこと（臨床）が最優先されることに変わりはありません。

Part 4: Learning Medical Expressions

Chapter 11 Expressions to Describe Pain

> **POINT** ☞ 患者さんが医療サービスを求める理由の中で最も頻度が高く重要な症状である「痛み」「疼痛」の英語表現を学びましょう。

Reading

A suspected case of angina pectoris

(Mr. Kerr is visiting his family doctor.)

Mr. Kerr: When I was lifting a heavy box last night, my chest started aching.

Doctor: How long did the pain last?

Mr. Kerr: Well, my chest pain went away soon after I got some rest.

Doctor: Do you feel any pain right now?

Mr. Kerr: No, not at all. I'm pain-free now. The pain subsided immediately after I stopped lifting things. It completely disappeared within a couple of minutes. I guess it lasted only 5 minutes or so.

Doctor: Well, could you show me exactly where it hurt last night?

Mr. Kerr: Right across here in my chest, Doc. It was just under my breast bone.

Doctor: Have you ever experienced this kind of chest pain before?

Mr. Kerr: Yes, I have. Actually this was the third time this month.

COLUMN

「痛み」の表現

　患者さんが医師を訪れる主たる理由は何でしょうか？ 学校・職場健診，住民健診あるいは人間ドックなどで何らかの異状を指摘されたために受診するでしょうか？ 確かにそういうケースもあるでしょうが，実際には，患者さんの多くは「痛み」に関連した症状を持ち，それに伴う「不安」を心に秘めながら医療機関を受診してくることが多いのです。「痛み」を客観的に測定できる装置はないし，患者さんにしかわからないこの主観的「痛み」というものを，医師はできるだけ正確に理解するようにしなければなりません。この章では「痛み」についての口語的表現や語彙を中心に学びます。

日本語訳

狭心症が疑われる症例

（カー氏がかかりつけ医を訪れている。）

患者：昨夜，重い箱を持ち上げていたとき，胸が痛くなってきました。

医師：痛みはどれくらい続きましたか？

患者：胸の痛みは，ちょっと休んだらすぐによくなってしまいました。

医師：今はもう全然痛みを感じてないのですね。

患者：全然痛みはありません。持ち上げていた物を下ろしたら，すぐに痛みも弱くなってきました。そして数分以内に全然痛くなくなりました。おそらく5分くらい続いただけだと思います。

医師：さて，それでは昨夜痛かったところはどこでしょうか。

患者：胸のちょうどここです，先生。ちょうど胸骨の裏側あたりのところでした。

医師：以前にも同じような胸痛を経験したことはありますか？

患者：ええ，あります。実際のところ今回のが今月3回目の胸痛だったのです。

Doctor: When did you first notice your chest pain?

Mr. Kerr: I had the first chest pain 3 months ago when I was jogging. At first I thought it was nothing because my chest pain had always gone away within a couple of minutes after I stopped strenuous activities. But I started worrying about it as a friend died of a heart attack last month.

Doctor: I see. Tell me more about your chest pain. What kind of pain was it?

Mr. Kerr: Well, most of the time it was a squeezing pain or a pressing feeling in the center of my chest. Sometimes it would spread to my left shoulder.

Doctor: At this stage, I would like to take a look at you. Let me listen to your chest. So could you just strip to the waist please?

After the physical examination:

Doctor: Nothing wrong with your physical examination. At this point, we are not sure of the diagnosis. But based on what you described to me, the diagnosis would appear to be angina. We need some tests to make a definite diagnosis. So let's schedule an ECG and a treadmill stress test and see what's going on.

医師：初めて胸痛に気付いたのはいつですか？

患者：3ヵ月前にジョギング中に初めて胸痛を自覚しました。最初はその胸痛が激しい運動をやめて2〜3分すると完全に消えるので，あまり気にしていませんでした。しかし，友人の一人が先月心臓発作で亡くなったこともあって，気になりはじめました。

医師：なるほど，わかりました。胸痛についてもっと詳しくお話ください。どんな種類の痛みでしたか？

患者：そうですね，ほとんどの場合，締め付けられるような，押されるような感じの痛みです。ときどき左の肩に痛みが放散します。

医師：ではさっそくですが診察しましょう。胸を聴診しますから，上半身の衣服を脱いでください。

診察の後で

医師：診察では何も異常はありません。現段階でははっきりとは診断できませんが，これまでのお話からすると，狭心症の可能性が考えられます。はっきり診断するためにはいくつかの検査が必要です。心電図検査やトレッドミル負荷試験をやってみて，その結果がどうなるか診ていきましょう。

Word Check

■ 痛みに関する表現

- **pain-free** [péin-fríː]　痛みのない

  (名詞の直後に -free を付けて「…のない」という意味の形容詞をつくることができる。例えば sugar-free[砂糖を含まない；無糖の]，tax-free[免税の]などがある)

- **squeezing pain**　締め付けるような痛み，圧迫するような痛み

■ 基本的な医学用語・検査用語

- **angina pectoris** [ændʒáɪnə péktərɪs]　狭心症

  (一般的な発音は [ændʒáɪnə] であるが，心臓専門医[cardiologist]同士の間ではラテン語風に [ændʒənə] と発音されることもある)

- **family doctor**　家庭医

  (家庭医学を専門とする医師のことで，一家のかかりつけ医である。family physician ともいう。関連語彙として，専門医[specialist]に対して一般開業医を GP[general practitioner]とか primary care physician などという)

- **treadmill stress test** (= treadmill exercise test)　トレッドミル〔運動〕負荷試験

  (狭心症等の虚血性心疾患の確定診断をするために行う)

■ 動詞表現

- **subside** [səbsáɪd] v. 鎮まる，治まる

  (疼痛が治まるような場合に用いる動詞。【語源分析】subside → sub-(下に)＋ side(座る，定着する)→下方に向かって行き底で落ち着く→沈下する，落ち込む→鎮まる，治まる)

- **die of …**　…で死ぬ，…で死亡する

  ("…"のところに病名が入る。病気が原因で死ぬ場合は

ほとんどすべてこの "die of ..." という表現で間に合うが，死因が外傷の場合には "die from ..." とすることもある。例えば "She died from a trauma to the head." ［彼女は頭部外傷で死亡した。］）

- **spread to ...**　…へ広がる，…に波及する

（痛みが1ヵ所から他の場所へ放散する場合にもこの表現が使える。例えば "The chest pain spread to my left shoulder and then to the neck." ［胸痛は左の肩に放散し，次に首にも広がりました。］）

- **take a look at ...**　…を見る，…を診る
- **listen to one's chest**　胸を聴診する
- **make a definite diagnosis**　確定診断する

■ 会話表現

- **How long did the pain last?**「痛みはどれくらいの間続きましたか？」

（痛みがどれくらいの間持続したのかを直接的に尋ねるときの典型的な質問。the pain は患者が実際に経験した chest pain のことを指すので定冠詞 "the" を用いている）

- **Could you show me exactly where it hurt?**「どこが痛かったか正確に示してください。」

（疼痛の場所を尋ねる際の基本的な表現。「どこが痛いのか示してくださいますか？」は "Could you show me where it hurts?" フレーズとして show me where it hurts を覚えておくと便利）

- **Have you ever experienced ...?**「これまでに…を経験したことがありますか？」

（"..." のところに症状や病気などを入れて表現する。病歴をとる際に役立つ表現）

- **When did you first notice ...?**「…を最初に気付いたのはいつですか？」

- **Tell me more about your chest pain.**「胸痛についてもっと詳しく話してください。」
  (痛みについての情報をより詳しく知るためには，tell me more about ...［…についてもう少し詳しく教えてください］のような表現で問いかけるのがよい)

■その他
- **right across here**　ちょうどここを横切るように，ちょうどこの辺に
- **at first**　最初は
  (しばしば後に but を伴う。「最初は…，しかし〜」)
- **at this stage**　この段階で，現段階では
- **at this point** (= at this time)　現時点では，現段階では

Word Study

■「痛み」の有無を尋ねる表現

「…に痛みがありますか？」と尋ねる場合には，"Do you have any pain in ...?"（あるいは "Do you have a pain in ...?" や "Do you have pain in ...?"）が使えます。例えば「首のところが痛みますか？」は "Do you have any pain in your neck?" ということができます。同様に「しびれ（知覚麻痺，numbness）」や「チクチクするような痛み（知覚異常，tingling）」について尋ねる場合も，上記の pain の代わりに numbness や tingling に置き換えて，「手や足にしびれ感がありますか？」なら，"Do you have any numbness in your hands or feet?"「腕や脚にチクチクするような痛みや異常な感じがありますか？」なら，"Do you have any tingling in your arms or legs?" と表現できます。

豆知識

pain in the neck　医学的なこととは関係ありませんが，"pain in the neck" と言うと「目の上のこぶ」「悩みの種」「面倒くさいこと」の意味でも用いられます。例えば "Studying English is a pain in the neck" のように使います。また日本人は使用すべきではないでしょうが，実は "pain in the neck" よりも "pain in the ass" のフレーズの方が，日常会話でよく耳にする表現です。

Chapter 11　Expressions of Pain

「痛み」と一言にいってもさまざまな痛みがあります．その痛みの性質について詳しく知りたい場合には，"How could you describe your pain?"とか"Can you describe your pain?", "Could you describe your pain in more detail?"などと尋ねます．あるいはもっと簡単に"What is your pain like?"とも表現できます．

さまざまな痛みを英語で表現する際には，以下のような形容詞をよく用いるので，一通り覚えておく必要があります．

痛みの修飾語

英語	日本語	具体的な疼痛の例語
splitting	割れるように痛む	splitting headache（割れるように痛む頭痛）
throbbing	ズキズキ痛む	throbbing headache（ズキズキする頭痛） throbbing toothache（ズキズキする歯痛）
pounding	ズキズキよりももっとひどく脈打つように痛む	pounding headache（ズキンズキンと脈打つような頭痛）
band-like	はちまきで締め付けられるように痛む	band-like headache（締め付けられるような頭痛）
dull	鈍い，シクシクと痛む	dull headache（シクシク痛む頭痛） dull toothache（シクシク痛む歯痛） dull pain（体のどこでも「鈍くシクシク痛む疼痛」ならこれで表せる）
sharp	鋭い，キリキリ痛む，	sharp headache（キリキリ痛む頭痛） sharp toothache（キリキリ痛む歯痛） sharp pain（体のどこでも「鋭くキリキリ痛む疼痛」ならこれで表せる）
aching	うずくように痛む	aching back pain（うずくような背中の痛み）
colicky	疝痛の，差し込むように痛む	colicky abdominal pain（腹部の疝痛）
cramping	痙攣性の痛みの	cramping pain（通常は消化管に特徴的な痙攣性の痛み）
burning	灼熱感のある，ヒリヒリ痛む	burning pain（焼け付くようなヒリヒリする痛み）
squeezing	締め付けるような，圧迫するような	squeezing pain（典型的なのが狭心症に伴う締め付けられるような痛み）

■「痛み」の存在を訴える

「…に痛みがある」を表現するためには，"I have an aching pain in my lower back"（腰にうずくような痛みがあります）の例文でもわかるように "have a pain in one's …" の "…" のところに身体の部位を入れます。そして前頁の表に示した痛みの修飾語を pain の前に付けて，痛みの性質を表します。以下にいくつか例文を示します。（注: pain の前の不定冠詞 "a" を省いた "have pain in one's …" や代わりに "some" を入れて "have some pain in one's …" とする場合もあります。）

- ☐ I have a throbbing pain in my back tooth.
  （奥歯がズキズキ痛みます。）
- ☐ I have some pain in my head in the afternoon.
  （午後になると少し頭が痛みます。）
- ☐ I have burning pain in my feet and hands.
  （手足にヒリヒリするような痛みがあります。）
- ☐ I have pain in my ears.
  （耳が痛みます。）
- ☐ I have a pain in my neck.
  （首が痛みます。）
- ☐ I have renal colic.
  （腎疝痛があります。）
- ☐ I have biliary colic.
  （胆石疝痛があります。）

ところで「痛み」を表すのに "-ache" を語尾に持つひとまとまりの単語群があります。そこで，次にそれらを用いた例文を掲げてみます。

☐ I have a headache in the evening.

（夕方になると頭痛がします。）

☐ I have a splitting headache.

（割れるような頭痛がします。）

☐ I have an earache in both of my ears.

（両耳が痛みます。）

☐ I have a toothache.

（歯が痛みます。）

☐ I have a throbbing toothache.

（歯がズキズキ痛みます。）

☐ I have a stomachache.

（胃が痛みます / 胃痛がします / お腹が痛みます / 腹痛がします。）

☐ I have a dull backache.

（鈍い背部痛があります / シクシク背中が痛みます。）

COLUMN

さまざまな意味をもつ "colic"

colic には形容詞として「結腸の，大腸の」という意味もありますが，名詞では「疝痛」という意味になります。renal colic は尿路結石による「腎疝痛」であり，biliary colic は胆石による疝痛を意味します。

"Some babies have colic" というような文脈で使われる場合は，「痛み」というよりも，習慣的に毎日何時間かは泣き叫ぶ赤ん坊のことを表現しています。"My baby is colicky" などと表現することもあります。ミルクを飲んで，そのために腸が痛くなって泣くと考えられたのかもしれません。腸が非常に敏感なのでそうなるとも考えられています。"colic" と "colicky" は，小児を診る際には頭に置いておくべき単語です。

Exercise

1. 種々の痛みのニュアンスの違いを表現してみましょう。

   痛みの修飾語をまとめた 123 頁の表を参考に，以下の例にならって自分がその痛みを持っているとして①〜⑤に関して文章をつくってみましょう。

例：	頭痛	→	headache	→	I have a headache. （頭痛がします。）
	ズキズキする頭痛	→	throbbing headache	→	I have a throbbing headache.
	締め付けられるような頭痛	→	squeezing headache	→	I have a squeezing headache.
	ひどい頭痛	→	severe headache	→	I have a severe headache.
	軽い頭痛	→	mild headache slight headache	→	I have a mild headache. I have a slight headache.
	割れるような頭痛	→	splitting headache	→	I have a splitting headache.

   ①歯痛　→　toothache

   →＿＿＿＿＿＿＿＿＿＿＿＿＿＿＿＿＿＿＿＿＿＿＿＿

   ②胸痛　→　chest pain

   →＿＿＿＿＿＿＿＿＿＿＿＿＿＿＿＿＿＿＿＿＿＿＿＿

   ③腹痛　→　abdominal pain

   →＿＿＿＿＿＿＿＿＿＿＿＿＿＿＿＿＿＿＿＿＿＿＿＿

   ④腰痛　→　lower back pain

   →＿＿＿＿＿＿＿＿＿＿＿＿＿＿＿＿＿＿＿＿＿＿＿＿

   ⑤疝痛　→　colic

   →＿＿＿＿＿＿＿＿＿＿＿＿＿＿＿＿＿＿＿＿＿＿＿＿

2. 下記に示すような種々の痛みの性状表現 a)〜h) があるが，下に示す体の部分①〜⑧について，それぞれに特徴的な痛みを表現するのにふさわしい疼痛の種類を a 〜 h から選びなさい。答えは 1 種類とは限りません。

a) cramping pain　　　b) splitting pain　　　c) throbbing pain
d) aching pain　　　　e) sharp pain　　　　f) colicky pain
g) stabbing pain　　　h) squeezing pain

① back　　　　　　　　→ (　　　)
② head　　　　　　　　→ (　　　)
③ heart　　　　　　　　→ (　　　)
④ abdomen　　　　　　→ (　　　)
⑤ tooth　　　　　　　　→ (　　　)
⑥ colon　　　　　　　　→ (　　　)
⑦ chest or abdomen　　→ (　　　)
⑧ appendix　　　　　　→ (　　　)

3. "Do you have any pain in your ...?" という表現を用いて，色々な部位の痛みの有無を尋ねる文章を少なくとも 5 つ書いてみましょう。

_____

_____

_____

_____

_____

4. 語尾が "-ache" で終わる痛みを表す単語をできるだけ多く書き出しましょう。

_____

_____

_____

_____

5. "I have a pain in my ..." (あるいは "I have pain in my ...") という表現を用いて，"..." に身体の部位を入れ次のような部位の痛みがあることを表現しましょう。

例： 頭の痛み → **I have a pain in my head.**

①首の痛み → _____

②肩の痛み → _____

③胸の痛み → _____

④腹部の痛み → _____

⑤骨盤部の痛み → _____

⑥背中の痛み → _____

⑦手足の痛み → _____

Chapter 11 Expressions of Pain

Part 4: Learning Medical Expressions

Chapter 12 Expressions to Use in the Examination

> **POINT** ☞ 患者さんが検査を受ける際に用いられる口語表現を学びましょう。

Reading

Case 1. A patient with bronchitis

Doctor: So, you've been coughing constantly for a week now, right?

Mr. Parkinson: Yeah, that's about it.

Doctor: Well, Mr. Parkinson, let me have a look at you now. Will you take off your shirt and lie on the couch please? First, I'm going to listen to your chest. Take a deep breath, ..., again. Well, the respiratory sounds are slightly weak. Now, I'm listening to your heart. Next, I'm going to feel your abdomen. Try to relax. Any tenderness here? ...

Mr. Parkinson: No, sir.

Doctor: All done. You can get dressed now.

Mr. Parkinson: Anything wrong?

Doctor: Well, Mr. Parkinson, you seem to have bronchitis. I don't think you have pneumonia and I assume this will clear up on its own. But just to make sure, I'd like to take an x-ray of your chest, an ECG, and some blood tests.

日本語訳

症例 1．気管支炎の患者さん

医師：それでここ 1 週間咳がずっと続いているのですね。

患者：ええ，そんな感じです。

医師：ではパーキンソンさん，診察しましょう。シャツを脱いで診察台に横になってくださいますか。まず，胸を聴診します。深呼吸してください。もう一度…。少し呼吸音が弱くなっているかもしれませんね。では次に心臓の音を聴診しましょう。次に腹部を触診します。力を抜いてください。ここを押すと痛みますか？

患者：いいえ，痛くありません。

医師：これでお終いです。どうぞ服を着てください。

患者：何か異状があるのでしょうか？

医師：パーキンソンさん，どうも気管支炎に罹っておられるようです。肺炎はないと思いますし，経過を見ていけば自然に治ると思います。しかし，念のために胸部レントゲン検査，心電図検査と血液検査を実施したいと思います。

Case 2. A patient with a sprained ankle

Doctor: Hello, Mr. Kim. What seems to be the problem today?

Mr. Kim: Well, Doc, last evening, I just fell and sprained my left ankle.

Doctor: How did you do that?

Mr. Kim: I fell and twisted my left ankle severely in an attempt to kick the ball while I was playing soccer.

Doctor: Please turn up your trousers so that I can have a look at it.

Mr. Kim: It's been swollen, compared to the other side. Even the skin color changed into blue.

Doctor: Does it hurt when you walk?

Mr. Kim: Yes, very painful.

Doctor: I'm going to feel your left ankle. If it hurts, just let me know, OK?

Mr. Kim: Ouch! It really hurts when you push on my ankle.

Doctor: All right. Well, probably you've just got a severe case of sprained ankle. But just to make sure there is no broken bone in there, I think you should have an x-ray immediately.

Mr. Kim: Will you fix an appointment for me?

Doctor: Sure. You can go to the x-ray department this afternoon at 1 o'clock. I'll arrange the treatment plan based on the result. Anyway, it is a good idea to take enough rest along with the help of a pain killer.

Mr. Kim: All right, Doc. I'll see you later.

Doctor: Okay. See you later.

症例2. 足首を捻挫した患者さん

医師：キムさん，こんにちは。今日はどうしましたか？

患者：実は先生，昨日の夕方，転んで左の足首をくじいてしまいました

医師：どのようにして，そうなったのですか？

患者：サッカーをしているときに，ボールを蹴ろうとしたら転んでしまい，ひどく左足首をひねってしまいました。

医師：診察できるようにズボンをたくし上げてください。

患者：反対側に比べてかなりむくんできました。皮膚も青紫になってしまいまいた。

医師：歩くときに痛みますか？

患者：ええ，とても痛みます。

医師：左の足首に触って診察しますよ。もし痛ければすぐに教えてください。いいですか？

患者：痛い！ 足首を触られると非常に痛みます。

医師：はい，わかりました。おそらく足首の捻挫のひどいのだろうと思います。ただ念のために骨折がないかどうか，すぐにＸ線検査をして確かめましょう。.

患者：検査予定を立てていただけますか？

医師：もちろんですとも。今日の午後１時に放射線科の「窓口」に来てください。その結果に基づいて治療方針を決めます。とにかく痛み止めを飲んで十分に休むのがいいと思います。

患者：わかりました。ではまた後ほど。

医師：ではひとまず失礼します。また後ほど。

Word Check

- **lie on the couch** 診察台（診察用ベッド）に横になる

    （ここでは on the couch で「診察台の上に」を表現しているが，"lie on the examination table" ということもできる）

- **tenderness** 圧痛

    （押したり圧迫したりすると痛みが生じるような場合，そのような疼痛のことを "tenderness" という）

- **bronchitis** [brɑnkáɪtɪs] 気管支炎

    （【語源分析】bronchitis → broncho-（気管支）+ -itis（炎症）→気管支の炎症→気管支炎）

- **pneumonia** [n(j)uːmóunjə, njuːmóunjə] 肺炎

    （【語源分析】pneumonia → pneumon（空気，肺）+ -ia（状態，病的状態）→肺の病的状態→肺炎）

- **a sprained ankle** 足首の捻挫

    （sprain は動詞でも名詞でも使われる。「足首を捻挫しました。」なら "I sprained my ankle" あるいは "I had a sprained ankle" という）

Word Study

■検査の表現

　診断に至るまでの「検査」は，1) physical examination，2) laboratory examination，3) diagnostic imaging (radiographic examination) の3つに分類されます。

1. physical examination

　本来は「身体的検査」と訳すべきですが，physical という形容詞に「身体の」という意味と同時に，physics（物理学）の形容

詞としての「物理的な」という意味もあるため，以前はそれが混同されて，古い内科学教科書では「理学的検査」と訳されていたこともありました。医療ではphysicalという形容詞が頻出しますが，そのphysicalが「身体的な」か「物理的な」であるかを意識的に区別することが必要です。

　physical examinationはしばしば医療者間ではphysical examと省略して使われています。狭義には「身体検査」としての視診，聴診，打診，触診などの検査手技を実施することをいいますが，広義には問診も含めて「診察」と訳されています。

　視診はinspectionで，語源的にはin-（中へ）+ -spection（見ること）→中を覗き込むようによく見て調べること，となります。聴診はauscultationで，aus（耳）+ cultation（傾けること）→耳を傾け傾聴すること。打診はpercussionで，per-（…を通して，…越しに）+ cussion（打つこと，叩くこと）→体表を通して叩くこと→体表を軽く打ったときの反響や振動から内部の情報を感じ取る方法，となります。触診はpalpationで，palp（手のひら）+ -ation（…すること）→手のひらを用いること→手のひらを使い触って調べること，となります。

2. laboratory examination

「臨床検査」と訳されていますが，具体的には血液検査や尿検査，便検査，喀痰検査，病理検査などが含まれています。また，心電図や脳波，呼吸機能を調べることも含まれます。

3. diagnostic imaging

「画像診断」と訳されることが多いようです。かつてはradiographic examinationと呼ばれていた部門が発展して，一般X線撮影（radiography）だけでなく造影検査やCT（computed tomography），超音波検査，MRIや核医学検査，PETなどの画像を診断資料として用いるような検査法がまとめて

diagnostic imaging と呼ばれるようになってきました。

4. 検査の手順

　検査の手順としては，まず physical examination が実施されます。その際には次のように表現することが一般的です。

　　□ Let me take a look at you now.
　　□ Let me have a look at you now.
　　□ Well, let's have a look at you now.
　　□ Well, I'll take a look at you now.
　　□ Well, I'd like to examine you now.

　あるいは be going to を用いて，"I'm going to examine you now" とか，単に "Well, I'll examine you now" と表現することもできます。
　状況に応じて，服を脱いだりズボンをたくし上げてもらったりしますが，その際には下記のような表現を使います。

　　□ Will you take off your shirt and lie on the couch please?
　　□ Could you please take off your shirt and sit up on the couch for me?
　　□ Please turn up your trousers so that I can have a look at it.
　　□ Would you just take off your clothes down to your waist?
　　□ Can you please take your clothes off?

　特に患者さんが若い女性などで服を脱いでもらうことに抵抗を感じるような場合には，次のようなていねいな言い回しを使ってもよいかもしれません。

□ It would help if you could possibly take off your shirt and sit up on the couch for me.

続いて聴診・触診を行います。その際には，下記のような "I'm going to ..." や "I'd like to ..." を使った表現がよく使われます。

□ I'm going to take your pulse.
□ Let's have a look at your eyes.
□ Let me feel your windpipe.
□ Let me check the reflexes in your arms and legs.
□ I'd like to listen to your chest.
□ I'm going to feel your abdomen.

患者さんに「…してもらえますか？」と指示するときは，単なる命令形の文章でも構いませんが，"Will you ..." あるいは "Would you please ..." といった表現もよく使われます。

□ Open your mouth and say "ahh".
□ Stick your tongue out for me, please.
□ Please take a deep breath, and hold it.
□ Will you straighten your arm for me, please.
□ Would you please stand up as straight as possible?

また動作の確認などで「…できますか？」と尋ねるときは，"Can you ..." を使います。

□ Can you raise your arm over your head?

physical examination を終えて次の検査が必要な場合，次のような表現で，患者さんに検査の必要性を促します。

- ☐ I'd like to take an x-ray of your chest, an ECG, and some blood tests.
- ☐ I think you should have an x-ray immediately.
- ☐ I think we'd better do some special tests to check out your hearing.
- ☐ I think we'll do some tests and take an x-ray to check out what's happened.
- ☐ I'd like to do some blood tests to determine whether ...

Exercise

1. 医師と患者さんの役を決めて，**Reading** の会話を動作を交えながら再現してみましょう。

Chapter 5 Body Parts

Index

A

abdomen 35, 112
abdominal 35
aching 123
acidophilic leukocyte 41
acute myocardial infarction 107
Adam's apple 34
adenoid 11
adrenal cortex 48
adrenal gland 48
adult tooth 44
allergy 11, 93
alveolus; alveolar 43
ambulance 109
amniotic fluid 57
anemia 11, 93
anesthesiologist 6
anesthesiology 6
anesthetic 11
anesthetist 6
angina(pectoris) 120
angioid 27
angiotomy 27
ankle 36
antebrachium 35
antibiotics 74
antigenic 30
antitoxin 11
anus; anal 45
aorta; aortic 40
aortectasia 28
aortopexy 28
appendicitis 11
appendix 45
arachnoid membrane 51

arch of the foot, the 36
arm bone 38
armpit 35
arrhythmia 112
arteriosclerosis 11, 25
artery; arterial 40
arthralgia 17
arthritis 17
articulation 38
asbestosis 18
ascending colon 45
aspirin 11
atrial 40
attending physician 6
atypical 69
auditory organs 55
auditory ossicles 55
auditory tube 55
auricle; auricular 55
auris externa 55
auris interna 55
auris media 55
autonomic nerve 52
axilla 35
axon; axonal 52

B

B cell; B lymphocyte 41
baby tooth 44
backbone 37
bacteriology 11
band-like 123
basal ganglia 51
basophil 41
belly 35, 112

big toe 36
bile 57
bleeding 92
blood 40
blood capillary 40
blood & immune system ... 40
blood pressure 106
blood vessel 40
body fluid 57
boil 92, 112
bone 37
bone marrow 41
bowel movement 88
bowels 112
brachium 35
brain 51
brainstem 51
brain specialist 7
breast 35
breastbone 38
brisk 62
bronchial tube 43
bronchiole 43
bronchitis 11, 134
bronchoscope 11
bronchus 43
burning 123
buttocks 35

C

calf 36
calf bone 38
calm down 107
canine 44
capillary 40

carbohydrate 11
carcinoma 19
cardia 44
cardiac 40, 44, 107
cardiogram 21
cardiologist 6
cardiology 6
cardiomyopathy 21
cardiovascular 81
carotid artery 40
cartilage 38
case 70
cecum; cecal 45
cell body 52
cellular 52
Celsius 108
centigrade 108
central nervous system 51
central retinal fovea 54
cerebellum; cerebellar 51
cerebral cortex 51
cerebrospinal fluid 57
cerebrum; cerebral 51
cervical 34
cervical vertebrae 37
cervix of uterus; cervix uteri 50
cheek 34
cheek bone 37
chest 35
children's doctor 7
chills 92
chilly 92
chin 34
cholesterol 11
ciliary body 54
clavicle 38
clinic 11
clitoridean 50
clitoris 50

coccygeal bone 38
coccygeal vertebrae 38
cochlear duct 55
colicky 123
collar bone 38
colon; colonic 45
complain; complaint 4
conjunctiva; conjunctival ... 54
constipation 89, 92
cornea; corneal 54
coronary artery 40, 77
costa 38
cough 92
coxal bone 38
cramping 123
cranial nerves 52
cranium; cranial 37
C-reactive protein (CRP) ... 77
crown 44
cutaneous 56

———— D ————

dandruff 57
deciduous tooth 44
defecation 89
deferent duct 49
dehydrated 74
dendrite; dendritic 52
dental pulp 44
dentin 44
dentist 6
dentistry 6
dermal 56
dermatalgia 17
dermatitis 18
dermatologist 6
dermatology 6
dermis 56
descending colon 45

deteriorate 69
diabetes 60
diagnose 62
diagnosis 107
diaphragm 43
diaphragmatic 43
diarrhea 89, 92
diastolic blood pressure ... 106
die of 120
diencephalon 51
difficulty sleeping 93
digestive system 44
diphtheria 11
discard 74
dizziness 93
Doc 109
duct of sweat gland 56
ductus deferens 49
dull 123
duodenum; duodenal 45
dura mater 51
dysmenorrhea 30

———— E ————

ear 34
ear bones 55
eardrum 55
earlobe 55
earwax 57
echography 108
edema 92
elbow 35
electrocardiogram (ECG)
.... 21, 108
electroencephalogram (EEG)
.... 108
embryo; embryonic 50
emergency room (ER)
.... 72, 109

enamel 44
encephalomeningopathy . . . 22
encephalomyelocele 22
encephalomyeloneuropathy 31
encephalomyeloradiculopathy
 31
endocarditis 21
endocrine gland 11
endocrine system 48
endocrinologist 6
endocrinology 6
endophthalmitis 30
ENT doctor 7
enteral 28
enterospasm 28
enzyme 11
eosinophilic leukocyte 41
epidemic 69
epidermal 56
epidermis 56
epiglottis 42
erythrocyte 40
esophageal 44
esophagus 44
examination 5
external (ear) canal 55
external auditory meatus . . . 55
extremities 35
eye 34, 54
eye doctor 7
eye matter 57
eyeball 54
eyebrow 34
eyelash 34
eyelid 34
eyetooth 44

──────── F ────────

face; facial 34
facility 2
Fahrenheit 108
fallopian tube 49
family doctor 6, 120
family physician 120
fatal 76
feces 57, 89
feel nauseated 106
female genital organs 49
femur 36, 38
fetus; fetal 50
fever 92
fibula 38
fifth finger 35
finger 35
first finger 35
first toe 36
flank 35
fluid 74
flushed face 93
foot 36
forearm 35
forefinger 35
forehead 34
fourth finger 35
frontal bone 37
frontal lobe 51
fundus of uterus; fundus uteri
 50
furuncle 112

──────── G ────────

gynecologist 6
gallbladder 45
gastoduodenitis 20
gastralgia 16, 88
gastric 20, 44
gastric juice 57
gastritis 17
gastrodynia 88
gastroenteral 89
gastroenterologist 6
gastroenterology 6, 20
gastrointestinal 89
general practitioner (GP) 6,120
genital area 35
genital system 49
geriatrician 6
geriatrics 6
gerontologist 6
gerontology 6
get worse 90
giddiness 93
gingiva; gingival 44
glabella 34
gland 48
glossa 44
glossal 44
glottis 42
groin 35
gum 44
gut 112
gynecology 6

──────── H ────────

hair follicle 56
hand 35
hangover 93
have a bad effect 90
head 34
hearing loss 93
heart 40
heart attack 106, 112
heart doctor 6
heartburn 88, 92
heel 36
hematologist 6
hematology 6

hematoma 19
hemiarthroplasty 32
hemorrhage 92
hepatic 45
hepatic portal vein 40
hepatoma 19
high blood pressure 112
hip 35
hip bone 38
hip joint 38
hippocampus; hippocampal 51
homeopathic 11
hormone 11
hot flash 93
humerus 38
hyaloid body 54
hyparterial 31
hypercholesterolemia 30
hypertension 112
hypogastric 20
hypothalamus; hypothalamic
   .... 48, 51

I

ileum; ileac; ileal 45
immigrant 70
immune system 74
immunology 11
impaired hearing 93
inadvertently 70
incisor 44
incus 55
index finger 35
infection 74
inferior vena cava 40
inflammation 77
inguinal area 35
inner ear 55
insomnia 93

instep 36
insulin 11
intern 6
internal medicine 3, 6
internist 6
intervertebral disk 38
intestines 112
iodine 11
iris 54
irregular heart beat 112
itching 92
It's killing me. 107

J

jaw 34
jaw bone 37
jejunum; jejunal 45
joint 38

K

kidney 47
knee 36
kneecap 38

L

lacrimal (lachrymal) gland . 54
Langerhans islands 48
large bowel (intestine) 45
laryngeal prominence 34
larynx; laryngeal 42
left atrium 40
left ventricle 40
leg 35
lens; lenticular 54
leptomeningitis 30
leukocyte 40
licensed practical nurse
   (LPN) 72

licensed vocational nurse
   (LVN) 72
lie on the couch 134
lien 41
ligament 38
lingua; lingual 44
lip 44
listen to one's chest 121
little finger 35
liver 45
lobar 51
loss of appetite 93
lower back 35
lumbar vertebrae 38
lung 43
lunula 56
lymph 41
lymph node 41
lymphatic vessels 41
lymphocyte 41

M

macrocephalia 25
macrophage 41
macula of retina 54
macular 54
make a definite diagnosis . 121
male genital organs 49
malleus 55
mammary gland 50
mandible 37
maxilla 37
medical care insurance 2
Medical Law 2
medulla oblongata 51
medulla of suprarenal gland
   48
membrane; membranous .. 57
meninx: meningeal 51

metabolism 11
midbrain 51
middle ear 55
middle finger 35
Ministry of Health, Labour
 and Welfare, The 3
molar 44
monocyte 41
morphine 11
mouth 44
mucosa; mucosal 57
mucus; mucous 57
muscle; muscular 38
musculoskeletal system 37
myelin (sheath); myelinic
 52
myocardial infarction 112
myocardium; myocardial ... 40
myoma 19

N

nail 56
nail plate 56
nape 34
nasal 42
nasal bone 37
nasal cavity 42
nasopharynx 42
national examination 3
nausea; nauseous 88, 92
navel 35
neck 34
nephralgia 16
nephritis 17
nervous 51
nervous system 51
neural 51
neuralgia 16
neuritis 17

neurologist 7
neurology 7
neuron; neuronal 52
neuropathy 25
neurosis 18
neurosurgeon 7
neurosurgery 3, 7
neutrophil 41
nipple 35
nose 42
nostril 42
numbness 92

O

obstetrician 7
obstetrics 7
occipital bone 37
occipital lobe 51
omphalophlebitis 29
oncologist 7
oncology 7
oocyte 49
oophoritis 27
oophorocystosis 29
oophoroplasty 27
ophthalmologist 7
ophthalmology 7
ophthalmorrhea 57
optic nerve 54
oral cavity 44
orifice of uterus 50
orthodontia 11
orthopedics 7
orthopedist 7
osseous 37
osteoporosis 11
ostium uteri 50
oto(rhino)laryngologist 7
oto(rhino)laryngology .. 7, 31

outer ear 55
outpatient department 3
oval window 55
ovarian follicle 49
ovary; ovarian 49
ovum; oval 50
oxygen saturation 107

P

pain in the neck 122
pain-free 120
palm 35
pancreas; pancreatic 45, 48
pancreatic juice 57
pancreatoduodenostomy ... 29
panic 106
paranasal sinus 42
parasympathetic nerve 52
parathyroid gland 48
parietal bone 37
parietal lobe 51
pasteurization 32
patella 38
pediatrician 7
pediatrics 3, 7
pelvis; pelvic 38
penicillin 11
penis 49
perineum; perineal 50
peripheral nerve 52
permanent tooth 44
phagocyte 41
pharyngeal tonsil 42
pharynx; pharyngeal ... 42, 44
phlegm 57, 93, 112
physical examination 89
physician 6
pia mater 51
pineal gland 48

pituitary gland 48
placenta; placental 50
plasma; plasmatic 40
plastic surgeon 7
plastic surgery 7
platelet 40
pleura; pleural 43
pneumonia 72, 134
pollex 35
polyradiculoneuropathy 23
pons 51
poo-poo 89
poor appetite 93
pore 56
pounding 123
practitioner 6
precaution 69
primary care physician 120
primary physician 6
prostate [gland]; prostatic
    49
prostatism 28
prostatorrhea 28
protein 11
psychiatrist 7
psychiatry 7
psychoneuroimmunology .. 31
psychoneurosis 25
psychosis 18
public health 69
pulmonary artery 40
pulmonary vein 40
pulmonary 43
pulse 106
pupil; pupillary 54
pus 57
pylorus; pyloric 44
pyrosis 88

Q
quadruple 80

R
radiologist 7
radiology 7
radius 38
raise a (the) red flag 75, 77
rash 93
rectum; rectal 45
red blood cell 40
regimen 61
registered nurse (RN) 72
renal 47
renal pelvis 47
reproductive system 49
resident 6
respiratory rate 106
respiratory system 42
retina; retinal 54
rib 38
right atrium 40
right ventricle 40
ring finger 35
roentgenograph 32
root 44
runny ear 92
runny nose 92

S
sacral bone 38
sacral vertebrae 38
saliva; salivary 57
sarcoma 19
scapula 38
sclera; scleral 54
sclerosis 18
scrotum; scrotal 49
scrub 74

sebaceous glands 56
second finger 35
semen; seminal 57
semicircular duct 55
seminal vesicles 49
sensory organs 54
serum; serous 41
severe acute respiratory
    syndrome (SARS) 69
sharp 123
shin 36
shin bone 38
shoulder 35
shoulder blade 38
side 35
sigmoid colon 45
signs 90
skeletal muscle 38
skin 56
skin specialist 6
skull 37
sleeping disturbance 93
small bowel (intestine) 45
smooth muscle 38
sole 36
specialist 6
specialize in 3
sperm 49
spermatozoon 49
spinal cord 51
spinal nerves 52
spine; spinal 37
spleen; splenic 41
splenomyelomalacia 31
splitting 123
sprained ankle 134
spread to 121
sputum 57, 93, 112
squeezing 123

squeezing pain 120
stapes 55
stenosis 18
sternum 38
stethoscope 11
stomach 44, 112
stomachache 88
stool 57, 89
streptomycin 11
stroke 81
subcutaneous tissue 56
subside 120
sudden death 76
suffer from 90
sugar-free 120
superimpose 74
superior vena cava 40
surgeon 7
surgery 3, 7
sweat 57
swelling 92
sympathetic nerve 52
symptom 88, 90
synapse; synaptic 52
systolic blood pressure ... 106

T

T cell; T lymphocyte 41
tail bone 38
take a look at 121
taste bud 44
tax-free 120
temperature 107
temple; temporal 34
temporal bone 37
temporal lobe 51
tenderness 134
tendon 38
tertiary 80

testicle; testicular 49
testis 49
thalamus 51
thermometer 108
thigh 36
thigh bone 38
third finger 35
thoracic vertebrae 38
thorax; thoracic 35
throat 42
throbbing 123
thrombocyte 40
thrombophlebitis 22
throw up 107
thumb 35
thymus; thymic 41
thyroid gland 48
tibia 38
tissue fluid 57
toddler 65
toe 36
tongue 44
tonsil; tonsillar 44
tooth 44
trachea; tracheal 42
transverse colon 45
treadmill exercise (stress)
　test 120
treatment 2
trunk 35
try to relax 107
tummy 35, 112
tympanic cavity 55
tympanic membrane 55

U

ulna 38
ultrasonography 108
ultrasound 108

umbilical cord 50
umbilicus; umbilical 35
upper arm 35
upper jaw bone 37
ureter; ureteral; ureteric ... 47
ureterolithotomy 29
urethra; urethral 47
urinary bladder 47
urinary system 47
urine; uric; urinary 47. 57
urologist 7
urology 7
uterine tube 50
uterus; uterine 50
uvula 42

V

vaccinate 11
vagina; vaginal 50
valve; valvular 40
vein; venous 40
ventilation 73
ventricular 40
vertebra; vertebral 37
vertebral column 37
vertigo 93
villus 45
viral infection 74
virus 70
visual organs 54
vitreous body 54
vocal cord; vocal folds 42
voice box 42
vomiting 88, 92

W

weight loss 93
white blood cell 40
windpipe 42

Index

wisdom tooth 44
womb 50
wrist 35

――― Z ―――

zygomatic bone 37

――― あ ―――

悪影響がある 90
顎 34
顎先 34
足 36
足首 36
足首の捻挫 134
足の甲 36
足指 36
アスピリン 11
汗 57
頭 34
悪化する 69, 90
圧迫するような痛み 120
アデノイド 11
アブミ骨 55
歩きはじめの子供 65
アレルギー 11, 93

――― い ―――

胃；胃の 44
胃のような形の 20
胃液 57
胃炎 17
医学研修生 6
異型の 69
医師 6
医事法 2
胃十二指腸炎 20
痛みのない 120
胃腸の 89
胃腸病科〔学〕 6
胃腸病学 20
胃腸病学者 6
胃痛 16, 88
一般開業医 6
胃部の 20
移民 71
医療保険 2

陰核；陰核の 50
陰茎 49
インスリン 11
インターン 6
咽頭；咽頭の 42, 44
咽頭扁桃 42
陰嚢；陰嚢の 49
陰部 35

――― う ―――

ウイルス 70
ウイルス感染 74
右心室 40
右心房 40
うずくように痛む 123
〔病苦を〕訴える 4
項（うなじ） 34
うろたえる 106
上乗せする 74

――― え ―――

永久歯 44
会陰；会陰の 50
腋窩 35
エコー検査 108
S 状結腸 45
X 線撮影 32
エナメル質 44
炎症 77
延髄 51

――― お ―――

横隔膜；横隔膜の 43
嘔気 88, 92
嘔吐 88, 92
横行結腸 45
黄斑；黄斑の 54
治まる 120
落ち着く 107

147

おでき ……………… 112	寛骨 ……………… 38	筋肉；筋肉の ……… 38
悪心 …………… 88, 92	冠状動脈 ………… 40, 77	
おとがい …………… 34	関節 ……………… 38	——— く ———
親指 ……………… 35	関節炎 …………… 17	空腸；空腸の ……… 45
親知らず …………… 44	関節痛 …………… 17	薬指 ……………… 35
温度 ……………… 107	汗腺 ……………… 56	口 ………………… 44
温度計 …………… 108	感染 ……………… 74	唇 ………………… 44
	肝臓；肝臓の ……… 45	頸；首 …………… 34
——— か ———	眼内炎 …………… 30	くも膜 …………… 51
外耳 ……………… 55	間脳 ……………… 51	クリニック ………… 11
外耳道 …………… 55	顔面紅潮 ………… 93	…で苦しむ ………… 90
回腸；回腸の ……… 45		
海馬；海馬の ……… 51	——— き ———	——— け ———
外来部門 …………… 3	気管；気管の ……… 42	毛穴 ……………… 56
顔；顔の ………… 34	気管支；気管支の … 43	脛骨 ……………… 38
下顎骨 …………… 37	気管支炎 ……… 11, 134	警鐘を鳴らす …… 75, 77
踵 ………………… 36	気管支鏡 …………… 11	形成外科〔学〕 ……… 7
蝸牛管 …………… 55	キヌタ骨 …………… 55	形成外科医 ………… 7
顎 ………………… 34	きびきびした ……… 62	経腸的な …………… 28
拡張期血圧 ……… 106	救急救命室 …… 72, 109	頸椎 ……………… 37
確定診断する …… 121	救急車 …………… 109	頸動脈 …………… 40
角膜；角膜の ……… 54	急性心筋梗塞 …… 107	頸部の …………… 34
下行結腸 ………… 45	強膜；強膜の ……… 54	痙攣性の痛みの … 123
重ねる ……………… 74	恐慌 ……………… 106	外科〔学〕 ………… 3, 7
下肢 ……………… 35	頬骨 ……………… 37	外科医 ……………… 7
下垂体 …………… 48	狭窄〔症〕 …………… 18	下痢 …………… 89, 92
肩 ………………… 35	狭心症 ………… 79, 120	健康保険 …………… 2
活発な …………… 62	橋 ………………… 51	研修医 ……………… 6
家庭医 ………… 6, 120	胸〔部〕；胸〔部〕の … 35, 38	血圧 ……………… 106
下腹部の ………… 20	胸郭 …………… 35, 38	血液 ……………… 40
かゆみ …………… 92	胸骨 ……………… 38	血液〔病〕学 ………… 6
癌；癌腫 …………… 19	胸腺；胸腺の ……… 41	血液〔病〕学者 ……… 6
眼科〔学〕 …………… 7	胸椎 ……………… 38	血液・免疫系 ……… 40
眼科医 ……………… 7	胸痛 ……………… 106	血管 ……………… 40
感覚器官 ………… 54	胸膜；胸膜の ……… 43	血管切開〔術〕 ……… 27
肝癌 ……………… 19	キリキリ痛む ……… 123	血管様の …………… 27
換気 ……………… 73	筋骨たくましい …… 38	血腫 ……………… 19
眼球 ……………… 54	筋骨格系 ………… 37	血小板 …………… 40
眼瞼 ……………… 34	筋腫 ……………… 19	血清；血清の ……… 41

Index

血栓静脈炎 22	腰 35	耳管 55
血漿；血漿の 40	ごしごしこすって洗う 74	子宮；子宮の 50
月経困難症 30	鼓室 55	子宮口 50
結腸；結腸の 45	骨格筋 38	子宮底 50
結膜；結膜の 54	国家試験 3	子宮頸 50
腱 38	骨髄 41	軸索；軸索の 52
肩甲骨 38	骨粗鬆症 11	シクシクと痛む 123
検査 5	骨盤；骨盤の 38	耳垢 57
犬歯 44	鼓膜 55	歯根 44
	こめかみ 34	四肢 35
こ	小指 35	視床 51
好塩基球 41	コレステロール 11	視床下部；視床下部の .48, 51
口蓋垂 42		耳小骨 55
硬化症 18	**さ**	視神経 54
睾丸 49	細気管支 43	歯髄 44
交感神経 52	細菌学 11	鎮まる 120
口腔 44	臍静脈炎 29	施設 2
高血圧〔症〕 112	臍帯 50	舌；舌の 44
抗原性の 30	細胞の 52	下大静脈 40
高コレステロール血〔症〕..30	細胞体 52	膝蓋骨 38
虹彩 54	鎖骨 38	シナプス；シナプスの 52
好酸球 41	差し込むように痛む 123	歯肉；歯肉の 44
公衆衛生 69	左心室 40	…で死ぬ 120
甲状腺 48	左心房 40	耳鼻咽喉科〔学〕 7, 31
抗生物質 74	寒気 92	耳鼻咽喉科医 7
厚生労働省 3	産科〔学〕 7	しびれ 92
酵素 11	産科医 7	ジフテリア 11
好中球 41	酸素飽和度 107	…で死亡する 120
喉頭；喉頭の 42	三半規管 55	締め付けるような痛み 120, 123
喉頭蓋 42		尺骨 38
喉頭隆起 34	**し**	灼熱感のある 123
後頭骨 37	趾 36	収縮期血圧 106
後頭葉 51	C反応性蛋白 77	重症急性呼吸器症候群 69
抗毒素 11	歯科〔学〕 6	十二指腸；十二指腸の 45
硬膜 51	歯科医 6	絨毛 45
肛門；肛門の 45	耳介；耳介の 55	主治医 6
股関節 38	歯科矯正学 11	手掌 35
呼吸器系 42	視覚器官 54	樹状突起；樹状突起の 52
呼吸数 106	歯冠 44	

149

出血 ………………… 92	神経質な ……………… 51	頭蓋骨 ………………… 37
腫瘍学 …………………… 7	神経症 ………………… 18	ズキズキ痛む ………… 123
腫瘍学者 ………………… 7	神経障害 ……………… 25	脛 ……………………… 36
消化器系 ……………… 44	神経単位 ……………… 52	ストレプトマイシン …… 11
上顎骨 ………………… 37	神経痛 ………………… 16	鋭い …………………… 123
松果体 ………………… 48	神経内科〔学〕 ………… 7	
上行結腸 ……………… 45	神経内科医 ……………… 7	——— せ ———
硝子体 ………………… 54	神経病質 ……………… 25	精液；精液の ………… 57
症状 …………………… 88	診察 …………………… 5	精管 …………………… 49
上大静脈 ……………… 40	診察台（診察用ベッド）に横に	整形外科〔学〕 ………… 7
小腸 …………………… 45	なる ……………… 134	整形外科医 ……………… 7
小児科〔学〕 ………… 3, 7	心室の ………………… 40	生殖器系 ……………… 49
小児科医 ………………… 7	心臓；心臓の … 40, 44, 107	精子 …………………… 49
小脳；小脳の ………… 51	腎臓；腎臓の ………… 47	精神科〔学〕 …………… 7
上皮小体 ……………… 48	心臓〔病〕学 …………… 6	精神科医 ………………… 7
上皮性の ……………… 56	心臓〔病〕学者 ………… 6	精神神経症 …………… 25
静脈；静脈の ………… 40	心臓血管の …………… 81	精神神経免疫学 ……… 31
睫毛 …………………… 34	心臓専門医 ……………… 6	精神病 ………………… 18
症例 …………………… 70	腎臓痛 ………………… 16	精巣；精巣の ………… 49
上腕 …………………… 35	心臓発作 ………… 106, 112	声帯 …………………… 42
上腕骨 ………………… 38	靭帯 …………………… 38	精嚢 …………………… 49
食細胞 ………………… 41	身体検査（＝診察）…… 89	声門 …………………… 42
食道；食道の ………… 44	診断 …………………… 107	咳 ……………………… 92
食欲不振 ……………… 93	診断する ……………… 62	脊髄；脊髄の ………… 37
女性生殖器 …………… 49	心電図 …………… 21, 108	脊髄神経 ……………… 52
処置 …………………… 2	心内膜炎 ……………… 21	脊柱；脊柱の ………… 37
処分する ……………… 74	心拍〔動〕曲線 ……… 21	脊椎の ………………… 37
自律神経 ……………… 52	真皮；真皮の ………… 56	石綿症 ………………… 18
腎盂 …………………… 47	心房の ………………… 40	赤血球 ………………… 40
腎炎 …………………… 17		接合〔部〕 …………… 52
新型肺炎 ……………… 69	——— す ———	切歯 …………………… 44
心筋；心筋の ………… 40	膵液 …………………… 57	摂氏…度 ……………… 108
心筋梗塞 ……………… 112	髄液 …………………… 57	設備 …………………… 2
心筋症 ………………… 21	膵十二指腸吻合〔術〕 … 29	背骨 …………………… 37
神経〔科〕学 …………… 7	髄鞘 …………………… 52	前額部 ………………… 34
神経〔科〕学者 ………… 7	水晶体；水晶体の …… 54	仙骨 …………………… 38
神経の ………………… 51	膵臓；膵臓の ……… 45, 48	…を専攻する …………… 3
神経炎 ………………… 17	髄膜；髄膜の ………… 51	仙椎 …………………… 38
神経系 ………………… 51	頭蓋の ………………… 37	疝痛の ………………… 123

前庭窓 55
前頭骨 37
前頭葉 51
専門医 6
前立腺；前立腺の 49
前立腺症 28
前立腺漏 28
前腕 35

——— そ ———
象牙質 44
爪板 56
掻痒 92
足底 36
側頭の 34
側頭骨 37
側頭部 34
側頭葉 51
鼠径部 35
組織液 57
卒中 81

——— た ———
体液 57, 74
体温 107
体温計 108
胎芽 50
体幹 35
大臼歯 44
第3の 80
体肢 38
体重減少 93
大腿 36
大腿骨 38
胎児；胎児の 50
代謝 11
大腸 45
大頭蓋症 25
大動脈；大動脈の 40

大動脈拡張〔症〕 28
大動脈胸骨固定術 28
大脳；大脳の 51
大脳基底膜 51
大脳皮質 51
胎盤；胎盤の 50
大便 57, 89
唾液；唾液の 57
脱水した 74
多発〔神経〕根神経障害 23
卵形の 50
痰 57, 93, 112
単〔核〕球 41
胆汁 57
炭水化物 11
男性生殖器 49
断続的に 90
担当医 6
胆嚢 45
蛋白 11

——— ち ———
致死性の 76
腟；腟の 50
致命的な 76
注意 69
中耳 55
中心窩 54
虫垂 45
虫垂炎 11
中枢神経系 52
中脳 51
腸 112
超音波 108
超音波検査 108
聴覚器官 55
腸痙攣 28
徴候 88
聴診器 11

腸内の 28
直腸；直腸の 45
治療 2

——— つ ———
椎間〔円〕板 38
椎骨 37
ツチ骨 55
土踏まず 36
爪 56

——— て ———
低温殺菌 32
T細胞 41
手 35
できもの 92
手首 35
てのひら 35
臀部 35

——— と ———
瞳孔；瞳孔の 54
橈骨 38
同種療法の 11
頭頂骨 37
頭頂葉 51
動脈；動脈の 40
動脈下の 31
動脈硬化〔症〕 11, 25
突然死 76
トレッドミル〔運動〕負荷試験
.... 120

——— な ———
内科〔学〕 3, 6
内科医 6
内耳 55
内分泌〔学〕 6
内分泌学者 6

内分泌系 ………………… 48	脳脊髄瘤 ……………… 22	膝 ………………………… 36
内分泌腺 ………………… 11	喉仏 ……………………… 34	肘 ………………………… 35
中指 ……………………… 35		〔皮〕脂腺 ……………… 56
…で悩む ………………… 90	──── は ────	皮疹 ……………………… 93
軟骨 ……………………… 38	歯 ………………………… 44	脾臓 ……………………… 41
軟膜 ……………………… 51	胚；胚の ……………… 50	尾椎 ……………………… 38
軟膜炎 …………………… 30	肺；肺の ……………… 43	非定形の ……………… 69
難聴 ……………………… 93	肺炎 ………………… 72, 134	額 ………………………… 34
	廃棄する ……………… 74	人さし指 ……………… 35
──── に ────	肺静脈 …………………… 40	泌尿器科〔学〕 ………… 7
肉腫 ……………………… 19	肺動脈 …………………… 40	泌尿器科医 ……………… 7
二の腕 …………………… 35	排便 ……………………… 88	泌尿器系 ……………… 47
鈍い ……………………… 123	肺胞；肺胞の ………… 43	皮膚；皮膚の ………… 56
乳歯 ……………………… 44	吐き気 ……………… 88, 92	皮膚炎 …………………… 18
乳腺 ……………………… 50	吐き気がする ………… 106	皮膚科〔学〕 …………… 6
乳頭 ……………………… 35	吐く ……………………… 107	皮膚科医 ………………… 6
乳房 ……………………… 35	歯茎 ……………………… 44	皮膚痛 …………………… 17
ニューロパシー ………… 25	…に波及する ………… 121	表皮；表皮の ………… 56
ニューロン；ニューロンの 52	白血球 …………………… 40	病訴 ……………………… 4
尿；尿の …………… 47, 57	発熱 ……………………… 92	ヒリヒリ痛む ………… 123
尿管；尿管の ………… 47	鼻；鼻の ……………… 42	…へ広がる …………… 121
尿管切石術 ……………… 29	鼻水 ……………………… 92	貧血 ………………… 11, 93
尿道；尿道の ………… 47	パニック；パニックに陥る	
	………………… 106	──── ふ ────
──── ね ────	腹 ……………………… 112	副交感神経 …………… 52
粘液；粘液の ………… 57	腫れ ……………………… 92	副甲状腺 ……………… 48
粘膜；粘膜の ………… 57	半関節形成〔術〕 ……… 32	副腎 ……………………… 48
	半月 ……………………… 56	副腎髄質 ……………… 48
──── の ────		副腎皮質 ……………… 48
ノイローゼ ……………… 18	──── ひ ────	腹痛 ……………………… 88
膿 ………………………… 57	B細胞 …………………… 41	副鼻腔 …………………… 42
脳；脳の ……………… 37	鼻咽頭 …………………… 42	腹部；腹部の ………… 35
脳幹 ……………………… 51	皮下組織 ……………… 56	ふくらはぎ …………… 36
脳神経 …………………… 52	鼻孔 ……………………… 42	服を脱ぐ ……………… 134
脳神経外科〔学〕 …… 3, 7	鼻腔 ……………………… 42	ふけ ……………………… 57
脳神経外科医 …………… 7	腓骨 ……………………… 38	婦人科〔学〕 …………… 6
脳髄膜障害 …………… 22	尾骨 ……………………… 38	婦人科医 ………………… 6
脳脊髄神経根障害 …… 31	鼻骨 ……………………… 37	浮腫 ……………………… 92
脳脊髄神経障害 ……… 31	脾骨髄軟化〔症〕 ……… 31	不整脈 ………………… 112

不注意に 70
二日酔い 93
不平 4
不眠 93
噴門；噴門の 44

——— へ ———

平滑筋 38
臍；臍の 35
ペニシリン 11
ヘパトーム 19
弁；弁の 40
便通 88
便秘 89, 92
扁桃；扁桃の 44

——— ほ ———

膀胱 47
放射線科〔学〕 7
放射線科医 7
頬 34
母趾 36
骨；骨の 37
ホルモン 11

——— ま ———

膜；膜の；膜状の 57
マクロファージ 41
麻酔 11
麻酔医 6
麻酔科〔学〕 6
まつ毛 34
末梢神経 52
瞼 34
眉 34

——— み ———

ミエリン〔鞘〕；ミエリンの
 52

眉間 34
耳 34
耳たぶ 55
耳だれ 92
脈；脈拍 106
味蕾 44
…を見る（診る）........ 121

——— む ———

無糖の 120
胸 35
胸やけ 88, 92
胸を聴診する 121

——— め ———

目 34, 54
めまい 93
目やに 57
免疫学 11
免疫系 74
免税の 120

——— も ———

毛細〔血〕管 40
盲腸；盲腸の 45
毛包 56
網膜；網膜の 54
毛様体 54
もっと詳しく 90
モルヒネ 11
門脈 40

——— ゆ ———

幽門；幽門の 44
指 35

——— よ ———

養生法 61
用心 69

羊水 57
ヨウ素 11
腰椎 38
葉の 51
よちよち歩く人 65
予防接種する 11
四重の 80

——— ら ———

卵管 50
ランゲルハンス島 48
卵子；卵子の 50
卵巣；卵巣の 49
卵巣炎 27
卵巣形成〔術〕 27
卵巣嚢腫形成 29
卵胞 49
卵母細胞 49

——— り ———

流行病の発生 69
療法 61
リンパ 41
リンパ管 41
リンパ球 41
リンパ節 41

——— る ———

涙腺 54

——— れ ———

レジデント 6
レンズ形の 54
レントゲン撮影 32

——— ろ ———

老人医学；老年医学；
 老年病学 6
老年医学者 6

肋骨 …………………… 38

わ

脇の下 ………………… 35
わき腹 ………………… 35
ワクチン接種する ……… 11
…を患う ……………… 90
割れるように痛む ……… 123

　本書Chapters 6～8で使用する音声教材，ならびに各ChapterのExerciseの解答等をまとめた「教授用資料」を，ご希望の方にお分けします（ただし学校で授業の教材として利用されている学生の方は除きます）。ご希望の方は必ず**書面**（FAX，E-mailも可）にて，**書籍名・氏名・勤務先・送付先住所を明記**の上，下記へお申し込みください。

申込先：メジカルビュー社編集部　医学英語書籍担当者
　　　　〒162-0845　東京都新宿区市谷本村町2-30
　　　　　　　　　 FAX　03-5228-2062
　　　　　　　　　 E-MAIL　ed@medicalview.co.jp

講義録　医学英語 II

（担当編集委員：Nell L. Kennedy・菱田治子）

目次

Part 1: Reading Medical Features in News Magazines
- Chapter 1　What Is A Headache?
- Chapter 2　The Migraine Mechanism
- Chapter 3　Rethinking Treatments for the Heart

Part 2: Listening to Medical News Reports
- Chapter 4　Drugs for High Blood Pressure
- Chapter 5　The Battle between HIV and Antibodies
- Chapter 6　Drug to Stop Progression of Type 1 Diabetes

Part 3: Reading the Medical Research Paper
- Chapter 7　Entering the Medical Research Paper
- Chapter 8　Reading the Introduction
- Chapter 9　Methods・Results
- Chapter 10　Discussion

Part 4: Reading the Case Report
- Chapter 11　Case Report: A 33-year-old Woman with Abdominal Pain, Vomiting, and Erythema
- Chapter 12　Case Report: A 53-year-old Woman with Sudden Onset of Double Vision

講義録　医学英語 III

（担当編集委員：J. Patrick Barron）

目次

Part 1: Effective Communication during Medical Evaluation
- Chapter 1　Medical Interview and Medical History
- Chapter 2　Physical Examination
- Chapter 3　Diagnosis
- Chapter 4　Patient Information, Plan and Follow Up

Part 2: Giving Oral Presentation at Meetings and Conferences
- Chapter 5　Differences between Written and Spoken English
- Chapter 6　Preparing a Formal Oral Presentation in English
- Chapter 7　Taking Questions and Giving Team Presentations

Part 3: Writing a Medical Paper
- Chapter 8　Medical Writing: The Easy Way!
- Chapter 9　Commentary on the Uniform Requirements

講義録　医学英語 I

2005年 1月20日　第1版第1刷発行
2024年 4月 1日　　　　第18刷発行

- ■編　集　日本医学英語教育学会
　　　　　　清水　雅子　しみずまさこ
- ■発行者　吉田　富生
- ■発行所　株式会社メジカルビュー社
　〒162-0845 東京都新宿区市谷本村町2-30
　電話　03(5228)2050(代表)
　ホームページ http://www.medicalview.co.jp/

　営業部　FAX 03(5228)2059
　　　　　E-mail　eigyo@medicalview.co.jp

　編集部　FAX 03(5228)2062
　　　　　E-mail　ed@medicalview.co.jp

- ■印刷所　三美印刷株式会社

ISBN 978-4-7583-0407-8 C3347

© MEDICAL VIEW, 2005.　Printed in Japan

- ・本書に掲載された著作物の複写・複製・転載・翻訳・データベースへの取り込みおよび送信（送信可能化権を含む）・上映・譲渡に関する許諾権は，（株）メジカルビュー社が保有しています．
- ・ JCOPY 〈出版者著作権管理機構 委託出版物〉
本書の無断複製は著作権法上での例外を除き禁じられています．複製される場合は，そのつど事前に，出版者著作権管理機構（電話 03-5244-5088, FAX 03-5244-5089, e-mail：info@jcopy.or.jp）の許諾を得てください．
- ・本書をコピー，スキャン，デジタルデータ化するなどの複製を無許諾で行う行為は，著作権法上での限られた例外（「私的使用のための複製」など）を除き禁じられています．大学，病院，企業などにおいて，研究活動，診察を含み業務上使用する目的で上記の行為を行うことは私的使用には該当せず違法です．また私的使用のためであっても，代行業者等の第三者に依頼して上記の行為を行うことは違法となります．

講義録

■体裁　B5変型判，250〜850頁程度，2色刷り（一部カラー），定価2,500〜9,000円程度

呼吸器学
- ◆編集　　　杉山幸比古
- ◆編集協力　吉澤靖之，滝澤　始，吾妻安良太
- 定価　5,775円（5％税込）　　372頁

循環器学
- ◆編集　　　小室一成
- ◆編集協力　川名正敏，萩原誠久，中村文隆，吉田勝哉
- 定価　6,300円（5％税込）　　468頁

消化器学
- ◆編集　　　上西紀夫，菅野健太郎，田中雅夫，滝川　一
- 定価　7,140円（5％税込）　　700頁

内分泌・代謝学
- ◆編集　　　寺本民生，片山茂裕
- 定価　6,825円（5％税込）　　548頁

神経学
- ◆編集　　　鈴木則宏，荒木信夫
- 定価　7,140円（5％税込）　　568頁

腎臓学
- ◆編集　　　木村健二郎，富野康日己
- 定価　6,300円（5％税込）　　400頁

泌尿器学
- ◆編集　　　荒井陽一，小川　修
- 定価　6,300円（5％税込）　　352頁

眼・視覚学
- ◆編集　　　山本修一，大鹿哲郎
- 定価　7,140円（5％税込）　　384頁（全頁オールカラー）

運動器学
- ◆編集　　　三浪明男，戸山芳昭，越智光夫
- 定価　8,400円（5％税込）　　808頁

小児科学
- ◆編集　　　佐地　勉，有阪　治，大澤真木子，近藤直実，竹村　司
- 定価　8,925円（5％税込）　　852頁

血液・造血器疾患学
- ◆編集　　　小澤敬也，直江知樹，坂田洋一
- 定価　5,775円（5％税込）　　340頁

腫瘍学
- ◆編集　　　高橋和久
- ◆編集協力　樋野興夫，齊藤光江，唐澤久美子
- 定価　5,250円（5％税込）　　240頁（オールカラー）

産科婦人科学
- ◆編集　　　石原　理，柴原浩章，三上幹男，板倉敦夫
- 定価　8,190円（5％税込）　　520頁

医学英語 I
語彙の充実と読解力の向上
- ◆編集　日本医学英語教育学会／清水雅子
- 定価　2,625円（5％税込）　　168頁

医学英語 II
科学英語への扉
- ◆編集　日本医学英語教育学会／Nell L. Kennedy，菱田治子
- 定価　2,625円（5％税込）　　164頁

医学英語 III
専門英語の理解と実践
- ◆編集　日本医学英語教育学会／J. Patrick Barron
- 定価　2,625円（5％税込）　　272頁